Jump Start
Ketosis

Intermittent Fasting
for Burning Fat
and Losing Weight

Kristen Mancinelli MS, RDN

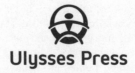

Ulysses Press

Published in the United States by:
Ulysses Press
P.O. Box 3440
Berkeley, CA 94703
www.ulyssespress.com

ISBN: 978-1-61243-835-1
Library of Congress Catalog Number: 2018944077

Printed in Canada by Marquis Book Printing
10 9 8 7 6 5 4 3 2 1

Acquisitions editor: Bridget Thoreson
Managing editor: Claire Chun
Editor: Shayna Keyles
Proofreader: Lauren Harrison
Cover design: Hannah Rohrs
Cover photo: © Daxiao Productions/shutterstock.com

Distributed by Publishers Group West

Contents

Introduction

In a world that seems so desperate for answers about how to get rid of fat, we seem determined to overlook the most obvious solution: spend some time not eating. In my professional experience as a dietitian, and my personal experience experimenting myself with weight loss strategies I recommend for clients, intermittent fasting is a very efficient way to lose weight. It's also very good for your health, and saves you a great deal of both money and time. If you can exercise, all the better. Fasting for weight loss makes so much sense that it seems almost unnecessary to write a whole book on the subject. And yet, you've probably heard these familiar adages:

"Breakfast is the most important meal of the day."

"If you skip a meal, your metabolism will slow down, and you'll end up gaining weight."

"If you don't eat every few hours, you'll be very hungry, and you'll overeat at your next meal."

"You have to fuel your body (with carbs) before your workout or you won't have the energy to exercise."

"If you don't eat every few hours, your blood sugar will drop, and you'll become faint and weak."

Most of us actually believe that something bad will happen to our bodies if we fast—probably because we have absolutely zero experience with it. But fasting doesn't make you weak, tired, mentally cloudy, or any of the other things people worry about before they try it. Nor does it slow your metabolism—actually, it does the opposite of all these things, for reasons we'll explore in great detail in the chapters ahead. Millions of people all over the world fast regularly as part of religious or cultural practices, and reap the benefits of improved physical health and emotional well-being.

But in our society, fasting is almost forbidden. The message we get again and again from nutrition authorities (not to mention every health and fitness magazine out there) is that the body needs small, frequent feedings throughout the day. Snacks are encouraged, and meals must *never* be skipped. As a result, we have literally convinced ourselves that we must eat all the time in order to avoid gaining weight. Does that really seem right to you? I find the idea absurd, and I think it has done a lot of harm to a lot of people. I suspect you're questioning it too, or else you wouldn't be ready to try intermittent fasting.

My goal in this book is to demonstrate to you that intermittent fasting is a very effective and safe way to lose weight—and specifically to lose body fat while retaining muscle mass. I aim to put to rest any fear you may have that skipping meals is bad for your body or will cause you to gain weight instead of lose it. I'll guide you with practical advice on how to integrate intermittent fasting into your life, and tips to make your fast go smoothly. I hope to have you so convinced of the benefits of fasting and the ease with which you can practice it that you commit to trying your first 24-hour fast before you finish this book.

If you've been fasting for a while then you already know that most people start out thinking they couldn't possibly do it and end up loving it so much that it becomes a permanent part of their life. If you haven't yet tried it and are worried about what it might be like (Won't I be hungry? Aren't we supposed to eat six meals a day? Can this possibly be good for me?), don't worry—by the end of the book you'll have read the personal stories of people just like you. People who thought they would never be able to go a day without eating, and who now practice all different styles of intermittent fasting that work with their busy schedules and life commitments—and keep them in the best physical shape of their adult lives. I believe you can start a fasting practice just as they did. If you are already a practiced intermittent faster and just want to expand your horizons, consider trying out a new fasting pattern while you read the book. With intermittent fasting, changing things up is encouraged!

In this book, you will also learn:

- Why breakfast is not the most important meal of the day, and frequent snacking can be harmful.

- How intermittent fasting enhances ketosis and ramps up the body's "fat burning machinery" to help you lose unwanted fat.

- How and when your body turns to stored food energy when you're fasting, and how to take advantage of that natural pattern to optimize your fast.

- Why blood sugar doesn't drop precipitously when you're fasting, and how intermittent fasting can protect against or reverse diabetes.

- Why fasting doesn't make you feel weak or lethargic, and why you can go to work, exercise, and do anything else while you're fasting.

- Why intermittent fasting paired with exercise can improve your metabolic flexibility, prevent your metabolism from slowing, and accelerate fat loss.

- What causes hunger, and how to manipulate your hunger signals to make your fast easier.

- How to eat when it's time to eat, whether you follow a ketogenic diet or not.

My Experience with Intermittent Fasting

I believe that by the end of this book, you'll have some days of intermittent fasting under your belt and will wonder how it was possible that up until then, you'd never gone a day without eating in your whole life. I believe it will happen to you, because it happened to me.

My first experience with intermittent fasting was in the summer of 2011. It was a deeply personal and (dare I say) transformative one, and I won't tell the whole story here—that will come later on in the book. For now, it's enough to say that the experience taught me something profound about what people need, and what we convince ourselves we need. The fast made me feel powerful and gave me a sense of freedom that I hadn't known was possible.

My second experience with intermittent fasting was for research. It was 2013, and I was living in Los Angeles (the home of many a great diet trend!) and working for a health and wellness company. My boss started fasting too. He was training for a muscular physique, and had heard talk in the bodybuilding world that intermittent fasting was a way to quickly drop body fat and build more muscle. As for myself, I was curious to know how intermittent fasting would affect my body and my hunger levels, and imagined I'd use that information later to help clients lose weight. We broke fast together every day with a light lunch at noon. I felt great—I didn't have to worry about what I would have for breakfast, and I had much more energy than I did when I ate in the morning. I quickly lost some fat in the belly area so that my jeans fit more comfortably. Plus, I love diet experiments, so I was having a blast.

At some point, I started eating breakfast again. As expected, I crashed most days around 10 a.m. when I should have been energized for a productive day at work. Some months later, I started the ketogenic diet and my energy crashes stopped. My curiosity was piqued. I starting reading more about ketosis, fasting-mimicking diets, and how to trick your body into burning your belly fat by avoiding carbs and limiting protein. I ate lots of fat and sometimes skipped meals, because I wasn't all that hungry. I lost the sweet tooth I'd had since childhood. My acne went away. My mood improved. I was able to concentrate at my desk for hours on end without losing steam. It was really remarkable.

I wanted to tell everyone how amazing the ketogenic diet was, so I wrote a book on it: *The Ketogenic Diet, A Scientifically Proven Approach to Fast, Healthy Weight Loss*. At the time, I was working as a dietitian in an outpatient program for adults, most of whom needed to lose weight and prevent "prediabetes" from becoming diabetes. I reviewed their diet records, and almost without exception, they began their days with a giant load of carbs: whole wheat toast with jam, oatmeal with dried fruit, yogurt and granola, a high-fiber bran muffin, and coffee with sugar or alternative sweetener. These people were not moving away from diabetes—they were speeding toward it. I knew a ketogenic diet and an intermittent fasting approach could help. I recommended high-fat diets, asked them to cut way back on carbs, and encouraged eating only between noon and 8 p.m. every day. I was doing the same myself. Although not everyone accepted my advice (some were afraid of fat, others just wouldn't give up their sugary breakfasts), I could see the more nutrition-savvy ones putting my suggestions together with articles they'd read about Paleo nutrition and the "good fats" in the Mediterranean diet, and moving in the right direction—even if they never fully took the keto plunge.

I found a ketogenic diet to be a bit too restrictive over the long term. After spending a few months on it, I wanted to expand my food options while still enjoying the benefits of ketosis for energy, mental clarity, and weight maintenance. I transitioned off a ketogenic diet to a more flexible low-carb plan (about 75 to 100 grams per day) and kept the daily 8-hour eating/16-hour fasting window. I have been recommending intermittent fasting to all my clients since, even if they're not interested in a ketogenic diet plan.

A Simple and Effective Solution

For any weight loss strategy to work, it has to be easy and convenient enough for people to want to do it. It cannot be too complicated, too expensive, or too restrictive. And that is maybe what I love most about intermittent fasting—it is simple to do. There are no meals to track, no calories to count, no macronutrient ratios to calculate. It's not only free, but will actually lower your food expenses. And it allows for moments of indulgence, enticing people to turn it into a lifelong practice instead of a lifetime of dieting.

I want to convince you that it's okay not to eat sometimes. You can go a day or two (or longer) without food and be perfectly well—and maybe even feel a lot better than when you're eating. The knowledge I share here about fasting, ketosis, and weight loss is drawn from my 12 years of practice as a dietitian, reviews of professional literature, conversations with colleagues who use these same weight loss tools with their patients, and interviews with experts in the field—as well as my academic training in chemistry and nutrition, and my personal experience with fasting and ketogenic dieting over the last 8 years. I believe there is something of a revolution underway when it comes to fasting and ketogenic diets and the recognition of the unique benefits these approaches offer in terms of reducing body weight and restoring healthy metabolic function. Where even a few years ago doctors were still asking patients to keep a low-fat diet and snack on carbs, today the recommendations are slowly starting to shift away from carbs and toward more fat for better health. Fasting is still on the cutting edge, and many more people are starting to embrace it for weight loss because they see the results. I suspect it is just a matter of time before the healthcare community at large discovers that high-fat, low-carb diets and intermittent fasting therapies are an untapped treasure and begins to use them again, as they did historically, to treat and resolve many more health problems—starting with the problem of excess weight.

I'll be honest, when I suggest intermittent fasting to clients their first reaction is usually, "Oh, I don't think I will do that." Then, with some soft nudging, and after hearing that I practice fasting myself, most of them come around to trying it at least for 6 weeks (my suggested minimum). Those that come to me already on a ketogenic diet are much more open-minded and will usually start intermittent fasting right away. A lot of people really enjoy having an intermittent fasting practice and love how it changes their body and mellows out their hunger. They appreciate that they no longer get irritable when it's been a few hours since a meal and can usually wait until mealtimes without snacking. Some people who have spent their whole lives listening to advice to never skip a meal try it, even though they just can't wrap their heads around making it a lifestyle. But even these people report how surprised they were that they weren't hungry all the time and could go a lot longer without a meal than they thought.

This book is for you if you want to explore intermittent fasting as a tool to lose or maintain your weight and want to develop new eating patterns to improve your metabolic health. It's especially for you if you want to train your body to burn fat for energy instead of glucose—a concept you may know of as keto-adaptation or fat-adaptation, or what you might see referred to on the web as turning your body into a "fat-burning machine."

If you're new to fasting, once you get into it and start meeting others who practice it, you'll really begin to ask yourself how it was that you ever managed to eat three meals a day plus snacks. You'll feel full faster, for reasons we'll discuss in Chapters 3 and 4. You may be amazed at how much less work it is now to prepare, cook, and find food when you have fewer meals to manage every week. And you will save the one thing all of us want and none of us can make more of: time. If you have gone on diets before and find yourself resentful that you have to do more shopping and cooking to prepare healthy meals, well, this time you're off the hook. With intermittent fasting, you'll trade in some of your body fat in exchange for an extra hour or more per day to do with as you choose. Not a bad deal.

This book is *not* for you if you are underweight, pregnant or breastfeeding, have a history of an eating disorder, or have any health condition that calls into question your ability to fast safely. Fasting may be problematic if you take any medication, so speak with your healthcare provider before changing your diet. If you are unsure whether fasting will be safe for you or you'd simply like more guidance on how to fast properly, seek the counsel of a qualified professional such as a registered dietitian or a physician—making sure they are familiar with fasting for weight loss. If you have diabetes and want to use fasting to get better, do not waste your time with a book. Contact Dr. Jason Fung and Megan Ramos at the Intensive Dietary Management program at idmprogram.com so you can begin fasting therapy to reverse your disease immediately.

People often ask me if I think intermittent fasting is a good "diet" for everyone. I politely tell them they're asking the wrong question—because when it comes to diets, as in *what to eat*, I can assure you there are many different healthy ones. You have only to look at the vastly different diets of people worldwide—from the Maasai people who eat only cattle meat, milk, and blood; to Hindus, Buddhists, and Okinawans who eat a mostly vegetarian diet; to the people of the Mediterranean who consume a mixed diet including lots of monounsaturated fat, fish, and some wine—to conclude that humans can thrive on many different combinations of foods. But intermittent fasting is not a diet. It's not a prescription of which foods to eat and which to avoid for better health. It's the recognition that human metabolism is built to deal with periods of feasting and fasting, and that constant eating breaks this system and makes us sick. Which foods you choose to do this with is of secondary importance.

I promote intermittent fasting because this strategy offers unique metabolic benefits that other "diet" regimens do not. I aim to show you in the chapters ahead why that is so, and convince you that whatever "diet" you choose to follow or combination of foods you choose to eat, that intermittent fasting should be a cornerstone of your health maintenance plan. That said, I believe lot of solving the weight loss puzzle comes down to what works for you as an individual. In my experience, more of it is practical than metabolic. So I will ask you to keep an open mind. Not everyone loves fasting at first, but a lot of people who come to it believing it will be difficult find that it's actually quite enjoyable. Be willing to experiment a bit, and try some new ways to organize your eating habits. Because if you're trying to lose weight without too much fuss or deprivation, fasting sure is a nice tool to have in your toolbox!

For my part, I've practiced intermittent fasting more or less regularly since 2013 depending on what I'm trying to achieve with my diet at the time. Professional reasons aside, as I approach 40—and with it, the prospect of fat gain and muscle loss every year if I choose to do nothing at all—I find that a low-carb diet, intermittent fasting, and varied exercise (no treadmills for me) are the best tools I have to maintain my body composition. I'm hungry less often when I'm intermittent fasting. My focus sharpens and my mood improves. I save a lot of money on food and fit better into my clothes. I enjoy the sense that very good things are happening deep down in my cells and DNA, probably lowering my risk of cancer and other diseases down the line. And I feel really powerful—like I can do something that I remember long ago thinking was impossible. I can go an entire day without eating, and it's no big deal! People think I'm so strong for it. I wish I could claim the credit! It's just the ketones, people.

CHAPTER 1

More Than Just Ketosis

Ketosis is all the rage. Since you picked up this book, I'm guessing you're on the bandwagon. You're in good company here! Maybe you're on a ketogenic diet or considering it. And if you want to jump start ketosis, then intermittent fasting is your ticket.

Truth be told, a ketogenic diet can be hard to maintain, simply because there are so many foods you can't eat. Even kale, the star vegetable of the 21st century, is only allowed in small amounts. I understand when clients say they're not up for the challenge of going keto. But I will tell you this: ketosis is divine.

Thankfully, if you don't want to do the ketogenic diet (or even if you do), there's a shortcut to ketosis—you can fast. Ketosis occurs when your body is burning ketones and fat for fuel instead of glucose. That happens in two situations: 1) no food is coming (fasting), or 2) few to no carbs are coming in (ketogenic dieting). When your body is in the fat-burning state, it makes lots of ketones in the process; hence, you are "in ketosis." It's completely normal for the body to be in ketosis, and it was certainly a common experience for humans throughout history who had intermittent access to food and periods of fasting in between. But the metabolic state of ketosis is very rare for anyone on a Western diet because (if I may speak for the crowd) we are always eating. When you're eating anything other than a ketogenic diet, you have effectively *zero* ketones in your blood. So it's quite uncommon for our generation of humans to be in a state of ketosis, unless you deliberately seek one out.

When you wake up in the morning after 8 hours of fasting, ketones levels are just beginning to rise. If you extend your fast until noon, ketone production will ramp up to supply some of the energy you need and your body will officially be in the famed fat-burning state of ketosis. Hooray! If you want to keep burning through body fat at a high rate, you need to stay in ketosis by sticking with your fast—for 16 or 24 hours, or a couple of days—and not by eating something ketogenic! There's a lot of attention on achieving ketosis with ketogenic foods, but if you're consuming keto foods, then where do you think some of the ketones are coming from? Not the fat on your hips and thighs. Fasting for ketosis ensures that the ketones fueling your brain are coming *only* from your body fat, thus getting rid of it. You'll learn all about how ketosis works in Chapter 3.

What Fasting Does for Your Body

Before we set our focus too narrowly on ketosis, let's consider the bigger picture. Yes, when you fast, fat will be burned and ketones will be made. But so much more happens when you're fasting—great things for the cells, tissues, and organs of your body, and some would say your mind and soul, too. If you have never fasted for even half a day in your life, then you may be thinking, "There's *no way* I can go 12 hours without eating!" But I am willing to bet that once you get started, you'll find it's a lot easier and way more fun than you ever thought possible, and you'll love it for a dozen reasons besides how quickly you'll lose your belly fat.

Fasting makes you burn through stored body fat when you haven't eaten for a while. You'll be burning so much fat that you'll be in ketosis. But fasting also trains your body to burn fat instead of glucose even when you're not fasting. In other words, fat burning isn't unique to the state of ketosis. Many cells in the body use fat all the time. The heart, muscles, liver, kidney, and other cells burn fat quite often. The trouble is that most of the time, while some fat is being burned, there's also new fat being made for storage because you're eating too much. Also, the cells that like to use fat rarely get the chance to do so for very long, because as soon as glucose comes in from a meal, they have to grab it instead. Too much glucose in the bloodstream is toxic, so it can't be left sitting there. So the priority for cells is to burn glucose first, leaving the fat untouched.

Most cells in the body can use fat directly for energy, no ketones required. But if you've spent a lifetime eating six times a day and you don't exercise at all, then they probably won't be doing that, simply because they're out of practice and you're out of shape. But they can. And that is really the end game when it comes to intermittent fasting: losing fat and building muscle while improving your ability to use both fat and glucose efficiently.

The ability to switch between the two main energy sources and easily use either fuel when appropriate is known as metabolic flexibility. If your cells are healthy and already accustomed to burning fat when needed, then intermittent fasting will accelerate your fat burning and help you lose much more of it by forcing your body to rely on fat as its sole fuel source. This is what people are talking about when they say the ketogenic diet and intermittent fasting will turn you into a "fat-burning machine." If your cells are *not* metabolically healthy and have trouble using fat for energy, then you need to exercise to prime the fat-burning pathways in your cells. So as you may hear a lot around the intermittent fasting conversation, exercise is important not so much for the number of calories it burns but for the fact that it improves the ability of your cells to burn both glucose and fat when they are available or needed. Metabolic flexibility allows your body to use the food energy you give it, in whatever form, to actually provide your cells with energy—instead of using it to bulk up your fat stores and leaving you tired and hungry as a side effect.

When the metabolic machinery is working right—when you've been intermittently fasting and exercising for a while—you'll be better at burning fat anytime. And you don't necessarily need to be in ketosis for this to happen, although you'll accelerate the process if you spend a good amount of time there, as you do on a fast.

If cells can use fat directly for energy, what's the point of ketones? Ketones are made largely to protect against muscle wasting during a period without food, i.e., an extended fast. Here's why: the brain is not as metabolically flexible as the other organs, and it can't use fat. The brain uses glucose when it's around, and the brain uses a ton of energy. So what happens when we don't eat for a few days and glucose supply is tapped? It turns out that humans can make glucose inside our bodies and don't have to eat it at all. But we can only make a small amount, and it costs us some valuable amino acids from body protein (muscle) to do so. We don't want to lose muscle when we find ourselves without food for a few days, because that would weaken our arms and legs and other important functions our bodies deem necessary for survival. So the body developed the neat trick of turning body fat, stored just for this very purpose, into ketones for the brain, without sacrificing other important things.

Voila! Ketosis became the thing everyone's chasing, the holy grail of fat loss. We're on message boards boasting about beta-hydroxybutyrate levels and posting videos of ourselves drinking fat coffee in the morning to put us into nutritional ketosis before a workout—after which we may just go eat a normal meal. We have "keto bread" and "keto cookies" (anyone else getting flashbacks of SnackWells from the 1980s?), and if you don't ask too many questions, it's easy to conclude that as long as you're in ketosis, the fat is just melting away.

Is nutritional ketosis a marker that you're in a fat-burning state? Typically, yes. Does that mean you'll be skinnier next month? Maybe. But how much are you eating?

Ketosis Doesn't Always Equal Fat Loss

A person on a ketogenic diet can have high levels of ketones and never lose an ounce if they eat too much. Granted, overeating while in a state of ketosis is hard to do, because one of the benefits of ketones is that they significantly dampen your appetite. But people do it. And I don't care what mix of nutrients you're burning for energy; if you keep eating more than your body can use, you're not going to lose weight. In an attempt to trick the body into thinking we're fasting, a lot of us gorge on fat. But we never consider what ketosis is meant for in the first place. Our hunter-gatherer ancestors did not have stevia-sweetened fat bombs or bacon-wrapped, cheese-filled burger bites or MCT oil shakes when they were in ketosis. They were in ketosis because they just had no food.

The reason the term "ketosis" even appears on the cover of this book is because it's the one that you know to look for—and without it, you wouldn't know that this book is full of strategies to help you train your body to burn more fat. Am I a fan of ketosis? Yes! But I urge you not to chug ketone supplements and drink fat coffee all day and expect to shed pounds of fat. Being in a state of ketosis *should* mean that body fat from your belly, hips and thighs is providing most of the energy you need. However, if you're meeting all of your energy needs with keto foods you're consuming, then the body won't need to turn to your fat stores for anything at all. If you're careless, or over-indulgent, you may net out on the positive side—storing more fat than you've burned!

If you're interested in ketosis and want to be sure that you're burning body fat instead of fat from your bacon breakfast, I recommend intermittent fasting. If you want to combine intermittent fasting and eat a ketogenic diet on the days you're eating, then go for it! Most of the recipes in this book can be used on a ketogenic diet, and we'll cover how to do it properly in Chapter 9. Remember, you don't have to follow a ketogenic diet to achieve ketosis through fasting. But even if you do decide to go keto, don't skip the fasting part. That is the really good part—and it's likely to get you where you want to go faster.

CHAPTER 2

The Unique Metabolic Benefits of Intermittent Fasting

If you think about it for just a moment, you'll realize we're meant to fast intermittently. That's what body fat is for—to fuel your body when you're not eating.

But when are you not eating? We're taught to eat three meals a day with snacks in between, plus coffee or tea with sugar whenever we're in the mood (or worse, soda or juice with every meal), and, for some of us, wine, beer, or cocktails to round out the day. And that's just a normal Thursday. On special occasions, we go out to eat at a restaurant and consume double-sized portions, and surely, we eat dessert. We eat extra at celebrations (no one is ever too full for birthday cake), or because someone brought bagels to the office (even after we've had breakfast), or because we received a gift box of chocolate (so rude not to accept), or for any other reason that sounds good. And a few times a year, holiday meals make even restaurant portions look meager, as we firmly believe that holidays are for indulging in so much food that we joke about unbuttoning our pants (or actually unbutton them) in order to sit comfortably after dinner.

Can you think of an occasion that calls for eating just a bit less in the same way holiday dinners give the green light to eat just a bit more? Ever heard of a holiday where everyone skips lunch? How about a national "underindulgence" day, where you take only small portions of food and leave some behind on your plate? If we have any of these, I haven't heard of them. I count the socially sanctioned occasions for abstaining from food to be the following: sleeping, taking a shower, using the bathroom, giving a presentation, and a few religious events. You might add "exercising" to the list, but I've seen enough people eat while exercising to disagree with you. We don't have nearly enough non-eating moments to balance out the eating moments. Most of our daily activities can be done while eating, and we proceed. We eat while working at our desk, driving to our destination, watching TV, relaxing at home, and so forth. We eat in between doing those things, if we feel like it. We simply don't take a break. If we snack after dinner and eat breakfast upon waking, our bodies get barely eight hours of rest from metabolizing food. All this overeating is making us sick, and there's no opportunity at all to balance it out—yet recommend that someone try fasting for weight loss and suddenly, you're an anarchist!

Of course, we know the nutrition party line. Eating small amounts at regular intervals throughout the day is the healthiest thing (so they say). It's not good for your body to go long periods without food (so they claim). You may have heard a number of arguments to support this recommendation, one of which is that you have to eat regularly to keep your blood sugar stable. This is absolutely untrue. The body has very tightly controlled mechanisms for keeping blood sugar stable. In a healthy person, the concentration of glucose in the blood is about 5 grams, and will stay within a very narrow range whether they eat a giant piece of cake with 50 grams of sugar (10 times what's in the bloodstream already) or go three days without eating anything at all. Blood sugar does not drop abnormally low in a healthy person when they fast. Keeping blood sugar stable is simply not a legitimate reason to eat frequent meals.

The suggestion that frequent meals will help control blood sugar and prevent weight gain is a dangerous one, because it actually does the opposite. Eating releases insulin. In addition to helping cells take up sugar from the food you've eaten, insulin blocks the removal of fat from fat cells and prevents fat burning and body fat reduction. And the more often insulin is asked to do its job of getting glucose into cells, the less sensitive cells become to its signal. Then, you have trouble using glucose for energy, and eating carbs further damages your health. We call that diabetes. But you also have high insulin levels, which means you'll have trouble using fat for energy, too, and you'll hold onto excess weight. This is how eating all the time breaks your metabolism.

A perfect solution to this problem is intermittent fasting. It undoes a lot of the harm that's been done from the frequent meals you've had all your life. Intermittent fasting prevents the constant stream of insulin from bombarding cells, and allows them to become sensitive again to its effects. Meanwhile, during your fast, as insulin levels fall, fats come out of fat cells and get burned for energy. This is how lowering insulin levels with fasting can produce weight loss, even in people who are insulin resistant, and prevent the progression toward diabetes or reverse the disease itself. We'll continue to explore the effects of fasting on insulin in the next section.

There are two other arguments in favor of the claim that eating all the time is a better approach than skipping meals. The first is that fasting will put the body in "starvation mode" and slow your metabolism, causing you to gain weight instead of lose it. The second is that fasting will cause you to lose a great deal of muscle mass in addition to fat. These arguments raise good points about the risks of dieting, and we'll discuss below why these concerns are unfounded when it comes to intermittent fasting.

Low Insulin Levels Allow You to Burn Fat

When you eat, the pancreas releases insulin into the blood, and a domino effect occurs. Let's think about what was going on before first domino fell, when you were in the fasted state, such as while you were sleeping. Upon waking up, your insulin levels would have been extremely low thanks to a long night of fasting. Fat from your fat cells would be fueling most of your body's energy needs, and you would just have begun to make ketones. If you waited a little longer to eat, then many tissues—including muscles, fat cells, and of course, the brain—would have been using them.

Then, you eat breakfast. Insulin levels almost immediately go up. Fats find their way back to your fat cells, along with some new ones coming in from the meal. They'll stay there for hours, until insulin levels drop again. What else is happening in the fed state? Assuming you've eaten some protein, the body will put those amino acids to use building new muscle, skin, or organ tissue, and other structures where they're needed. Assuming you've eaten some carbohydrate, glucose will be the body's main fuel source for the next one to four hours, and about a quarter of it will be stored in the liver and muscle for later use.

Insulin is what makes this all happen. It's the Head Hormone in Charge of energy use and storage. There are other players involved, but it's insulin that really runs the show. Insulin unlocks the door to cells and ushers glucose in. It grabs nutrients from the blood and stores them in fat cells. Assuming you've also eaten some fat with your breakfast, it takes three to four hours to be absorbed and stored away in your fat cells. This coincides nicely with the time that insulin levels (in a healthy person) take a good dive, meaning the hormone sticks around long enough to put away every last bit of food energy from your meal.

About six hours after eating, insulin levels return to baseline. You'd ideally move into the fasted state when insulin would stay low and the body would start to use fat for energy, keeping your weight nice and stable. But six hours of not eating? If you follow standard nutrition advice, you probably don't go half that long without having a snack! Certainly, by six hours after a meal, you're usually sitting down for another meal. If your breakfast was at 8 a.m., lunch will likely be at 1 or 2 p.m., and dinner at 7 or 8 p.m. Just when fat storage is slowing down and the body is turning to fat for energy, chances are, you're going to eat again!

But let's assume you've caught on to the benefits of intermittent fasting, and you don't eat again six hours after your last meal. Now, insulin levels are low. It's no longer blocking the exit of fat from your fat cells, and you can start to burn it for energy. If you fast until breakfast the next day, you'll burn up lots of fat—most of it toward the end of your fast, while you're asleep.

The fat burning will keep going as long as you stay on your fast. Insulin will only rise again when you eat something. Since insulin is really the "gatekeeper" that allows fat in and out of your fat cells, then you have to avoid waking it up if you want to burn fat for energy. This is why "grazing" or snacking is terribly counterproductive to weight loss. The goal is to keep insulin levels low and stay in the fasted state long enough to benefit from low insulin. While a 24-hour fast is great, you'll also get a lot of benefit from a 12 or 16 hour fast. If this seems way too much for you, don't worry. The hours add up faster than you think. And where are many ways to ease in to the practice, as you'll see in Chapter 6.

If you follow a ketogenic diet, then you may be wondering if all this applies to you. Fat, after all, doesn't cause an insulin response. The trouble is that even on a ketogenic diet, it's rarely the case that a meal contains pure fat. Even the most committed keto dieter doesn't eat pure butter or drink pure oil. Even bacon contains protein, as do other fatty meats, fish, eggs, and cheese. Nuts contain protein and carbs. Non-starchy vegetables like salad greens and broccoli contain carbs, too. So while the insulin spike from a ketogenic meal will be much lower than that of a typical meal, one shouldn't fool themselves into thinking there is no insulin at all. Two things to keep in mind if you are following a ketogenic diet and want to keep the insulin response low: 1) make sure not to eat too much protein, which triggers insulin release, and 2) do not "graze" all day on keto foods but rather keep distinct mealtimes, and extend your overnight fasting time before breakfast or after dinner.

Insulin Resistance and Weight Loss

Under normal circumstances, insulin levels should be low between meals and during a fast, and rise quickly to direct incoming nutrients to the right places when a meal is eaten.

Then they should fall again to allow the body to burn fat between meals.

But what happens if insulin levels never go back down? This is exactly what happens in someone who is insulin resistant. In this case, the cells become resistant to the effects of insulin over time and the pancreas has to send out more and more insulin to get the cells to respond. Eventually, so much insulin is required to get the cells to respond that insulin levels never really go back down. They remain high between meals, and rise even higher when a meal is eaten. Insulin is a very powerful signal to the body to store fat, so a person with insulin resistance will have a very hard time burning fat and losing weight.

Why Does Insulin Resistance Develop?

When your body is bombarded with a lot of something, one of the ways it deals is by lowering its response to that thing. Someone who drinks a lot will become resistant to the effects of alcohol, and as time goes on, they'll be able to drink more and more before they feel the effects. Caffeine tolerance works this way, too. Maybe you used to have one cup in the morning and feel jittery, and now you have two, plus another in the afternoon, and tolerate them fine. Some drugs can produce the same effect. Resistance is a healthy defense the body has to protect from the harm of excess.

Of course, we don't always take the hint that the body needs us to stop giving it whatever it's resisting. The drinker may just drink more, risking damage to the liver and other organs. And while coffee has some excellent health benefits, the example is still instructive: coffee in the range of one to four cups a day is okay, but you do not want to get so tolerant to its effects that you're lurching from cup to cup all day long just to feel alert. That's exactly what happens when someone with insulin resistance eats multiple meals per day or grazes all day long. The cells are exposed to insulin with greater frequency, and they react by becoming even more resistant to it. This just makes the problem worse. Resistance is your body's way of telling you that's it had more than enough, and it needs a break.

What happens if we remove the thing that's causing the resistance? If the drinker quits drinking for a while, he'll notice that his tolerance for alcohol goes down, and it will take a lot less to feel the effects. If the all-day coffee drinker quits coffee for a month, she'll find that she has become much more sensitive to the effect of caffeine, and it'll only take one cup to do the trick. In other words, the body responds to the absence of something by becoming more sensitive to it. So, to solve the problem of insulin resistance, we have to essentially "quit" insulin. But how can you quit something that's made inside the body?

You can stop doing the thing that causes the body to make insulin in the first place: stop eating for a while. Insulin is only released after a meal. If you skip a meal (or many of them), you will reduce the amount of insulin in your blood. Fasting is like a shut-off switch for the insulin production line in your pancreas: don't eat, and the machines stay turned off. Eat, and then eat and eat and eat more all day long, and the factory will be in full swing with no break in sight. In that case, insulin resistance will get worse, and when the body has finally had enough, it will progress to type 2 diabetes. In that case, the cells are so unwilling to respond to insulin that the pancreas cannot even make enough to force them to do so, and the person will need insulin injections—supposedly for the rest of their life (they may not need insulin forever if they get into fasting therapy, but sadly, many diabetics aren't told about this option). Of course, taking insulin injections makes it nearly impossible to lose weight, since one of the big jobs of insulin is to store fat.

But you can absolutely prevent this from happening by fasting. Intermittent fasting shuts off the steady stream of insulin, lets cells become more sensitive to its effects, and reverses the progression to diabetes and a lifetime of weight gain. If you have diabetes and are interested in fasting therapy, contact the Intensive Dietary Management program at idmprogram.com.

Growth Hormone Reduces Fat and Increases Lean Mass

Growth hormone reduces body fat and increases bone and muscle mass growth. Hmm...get leaner, stronger, and more resistant to osteoporosis later in life? How do I get this stuff?!

Growth hormone is, as you can imagine, very important in children because they are growing rapidly. We have less of it as we age, though it is still important, and is typically secreted during sleep. One of the functions of growth hormone is to break down glycogen (the storage form of glucose) to release glucose into the bloodstream when energy is scarce. Fasting increases growth hormone, which, in addition to providing the body with energy, helps achieve the goal of losing fat while avoiding loss of muscle mass. A typical low-calorie weight loss diet (which most diets are) doesn't achieve the same result. It's for its muscle-building, fat-burning effect that you may have heard of bodybuilders using artificial growth hormone to get leaner and more muscular. But artificial hormones can cause unwanted health problems, sometimes quite serious, and taking them is a risky approach to improving one's physique. Luckily, intermittent fasting does it naturally! Growth hormone, protein intake with your meals, and exercise help to preserve and build muscle mass.

Other things that stimulate the release of growth hormone are sleep (so it's good to get enough if you are seeking weight loss), exercise (ditto), and the "hunger hormone" ghrelin. Ghrelin is released to increase your appetite in the event that you skip a meal, and it also stimulates growth hormone. You'll notice it in bursts every so often when you're fasting. So when I'm fasting and I feel ghrelin telling me I'm hungry, I like to think that it's just there to tell growth hormone to build me nice strong muscles and bones, and I politely let it do its thing.

While new tissue is being built up by growth hormone, old tissues are also being broken down. But what happens to the old stuff? Good question! You see, the body does not keep all of its cells, proteins, cell membranes, and other parts forever. These things get old and worn out, and stop working properly. They need to be tossed out. In a sense, this is really what causes aging and disease—old parts piling up in cells and organs, clogging up all the machinery. Just as old knees and hip joints don't work as well as they used to, old liver and immune cells become defunct. So the body has mechanisms to clear out old parts that aren't working well and replace them with new ones, in an effort to keep things running smoothly.

One of the spectacular effects of fasting is autophagy (or "eating of self"), and it's the process whereby cells identify their own old and dysfunctional parts and destroy them, breaking down the structure and using whatever good parts are left behind to build something new and healthy. Suppose you have a smartphone that's glitching and you take it to the store to be fixed. You tell the technician that it freezes up when you open certain apps, the battery is draining too quickly, and the phone randomly shuts off for no reason. The technician uses some diagnostic equipment to identify which parts of the phone are broken, and then removes the old parts and installs new ones. The broken parts get disassembled even further, and perhaps the metal and electrical wiring that are still in good shape get transferred to a new battery whose other pieces were working well to begin with. Now it's got all the working parts.

Believe it or not, cells have that same ability to home in on what's broken and replace it with something new that works well, breaking down the broken pieces for energy when it's scarce and recycling the good parts to build new, properly working cellular components. But this process of autophagy is suppressed when a lot of new material in the form of nutrients is coming into the cell. In that scenario, there is pressure to build new components out of the materials coming in, and no time to devote to clearing out. So you are stuck with old parts as well as new ones, and things don't work as well as they could. During fasting, the body senses the absence of new nutrients coming in and triggers autophagy to begin the clearing out process so that, when you start eating again, there's a healthy foundation on which to build up new tissue. You can think of autophagy kind of like spring cleaning: if you never go through your closet and get rid of clothes that no longer fit, then anything you buy will just be crammed in to the space available—but if you set time to get rid of the old stuff, everything new will fit nicely into the space you've created. The body's ability to focus on clearing out old and damaged proteins during a time of fasting does a lot of good things, including helping the immune system to work better, derailing the growth of cancer, and preventing the accumulation of fragmented proteins in the brain that cause Alzheimer's disease.

So you can see how the combination of autophagy and increase in growth hormone really complement each other when you're fasting. Autophagy gets rid of out-of-date broken parts that are wearing the body down, and growth hormone builds up new tissues in their place. It's for this reason that growth hormone is reputed for its "anti-aging" effects.

Growth Hormone Deficiency

The importance of growth hormone in maintaining muscle and bone mass and decreasing fat mass can be well understood from considering what happens when growth hormone levels are abnormally low. Growth hormone deficiency is uncommon in adults and usually results from damage to the pituitary gland that produces growth hormone. Symptoms of this condition include a decrease in muscle size and strength, osteoporosis (a weakening of the bones), excess body fat (especially around the waist), and low energy levels—the opposite of what happens when growth hormone levels increase with intermittent fasting.

Intermittent Fasting and Your Metabolism

One of things most dreaded by dieters is the impact dieting has on the "speed" of their metabolism. (It's more relevant to consider energy expenditure, or how much energy you use that isn't formal exercise. We'll cover that in Chapter 5). When you eat less, as is the case with a low-calorie diet, you rob the body of some of the energy it's used to getting from food. To compensate, it uses less energy to perform basic functions such as metabolizing nutrients, maintaining body temperature, and so forth. The body conserves until energy going out matches food energy going in, and weight loss plateaus. If the person then decides to throw their diet out the window and increase the amount of food they eat, the body won't get the memo right away—instead, it will keep operating at a lower metabolic rate until it realizes that there is extra energy available and it can speed things up. But by that time, the person probably will have gained back all the weight they lost, and they'll be at square one.

Why does this happen? The body is smart, and it wants to match energy use with energy availability, lest things go haywire. Think about your computer. It requires electricity to power its processing activities. If you've ever been working at your computer and felt it get really hot, that was a sign that the machine was taking in too much energy and trying to get rid of excess by heating up. The body does the same. When too much energy comes in from food, it will speed up the metabolic rate by using more energy for its tasks, thereby getting rid of the extra it wasn't equipped to handle.

In contrast, say your computer is performing a lot of functions but isn't getting all the energy it needs. You're streaming a video online, you're trying to video chat with a friend, and your email program is open. The computer can't access more energy to power all these tasks, and it doesn't want to shut any of them down, so it just reduces the energy supply to all of them. The video slows down and pauses a lot, your conversation is full of delays, and it takes forever for the sentence you're typing to appear in the email on your screen. That's what happens to the body, too. If you consistently give it less energy than it's used to, it uses less than it did before and it slows the whole machine down, thereby slowing down your metabolism or reducing your metabolic rate.

Intermittent fasting doesn't produce this same effect because you're not sending the body a consistent message that there's less energy to go around and it needs to conserve. You're sending alternating messages of no energy, then lots of energy. When there's no energy, the body takes what it needs from your fat stores. Before it has time to reduce energy output and slow metabolism, you eat the amount needed to satisfy your hunger and put fears of an energy shortage to rest—so there's no need for the body to slow the metabolism. Keep this in mind when you consider your fasting pattern: it's best to switch things up. If you choose the One Meal a Day pattern and eat the same number of calories day in and day out, your weight loss is more likely to plateau. If you're at your goal weight and just want maintenance, that's great! If you want to continue to lose, you may have to alter the pattern so that you vary between a lot of energy intake (an eating day) and little to no energy intake (one or more fasting days). When you eat, eat to satiety. That means you won't hold back or try to restrict calories when you're eating, but rather will eat as much as you need to feel comfortably satisfied with your meal. This alternating approach to fasting and eating normally has a very different effect on the body than a diet based on a consistent, rigid low-calorie daily budget. It doesn't allow for the body to settle in to a cycle of low energy intake and low energy expenditure, followed by weight plateau, which most dieters dread.

The release of adrenaline during fasting may also play a role in keeping the metabolic rate running high. Fasting, like exercise, is a mild stress on the body, and produces many of the same positive results—increased muscle mass, less fat, reduced inflammation, and so forth. The hormone adrenaline is released during times of stress, sending glucose and fats from storage out into the bloodstream to give you more energy (presumably to hunt and kill an animal for food, because your brain doesn't know we have grocery stores now). Depending on the person and the length of their fast, adrenaline can increase energy levels and may sometimes even interfere with sleep. The good news is, between the ketones helping you focus and the adrenaline giving you energy, you'll get a lot done!

How Is Intermittent Fasting Done?

I am willing to bet that you've already had experiences with intermittent fasting. Have you ever had a day at work that was so busy, the hours just flew by, and before you knew it, the day was nearly over and you'd had nothing to eat? Or, maybe you've taken a road trip and remember that despite being hungry, you held off grabbing snacks at the gas station so you could make it to your destination and have the appetite to eat a nice meal? Have you ever spent all day caring for a child and been so caught up attending to their needs that you forgot to feed yourself? If you've done any of these, then you've probably clocked 8, 9 or 10 hours fasting.

Fasting can be done in short bouts that can fit into your daily or weekly schedule and provide great benefits. It doesn't have to be a long, drawn out thing. "Intermittent" means to occur at irregular intervals, beginning and ending again without a continuous pattern. That's exactly what intermittent fasting is. You choose the periods of fasting and eating that work for you, and you can adjust them as you go.

We'll explore many popular intermittent fasting patterns in Chapter 7. After you get comfortable with an intermittent fasting practice, you will create patterns that work for you. Some of the most common include:

Time-restricted eating. This means only eating within certain time periods. For instance, the 16:8 pattern means you fast for 16 hours (including while you're sleeping) and eat within an 8-hour window (6, if you can swing it). So you may choose to eat between 12 p.m. and 8 p.m., or 2 p.m. and 10 p.m. This is most commonly the "skipping breakfast" pattern, though you can have an early eating window and end your day with a late lunch at 4 p.m. if you choose.

Alternate-day fasting. Eat one day and fast the next day, alternating every day.

Intermittent fasting. Any combination of short periods of fasting. Some people do time-restricted eating every day and throw in one 36-hour fast per week on top of that. Some people fast on Monday, Wednesday, and Friday and eat freely Tuesday, Thursday, Saturday, and Sunday. You can do a three-day fast every other week. There are many patterns, such as a five-hour or even a one-hour daily eating window, fasting a few days per month, and so on. One of the best things about intermittent fasting is how flexible it is. Your goal is to alternate periods of eating with periods of not eating to elicit hormonal signals that tell your body to use stored fat for energy and keep your metabolic rate stable. You are encouraged to play around and adjust to find what works for you.

The next chapters cover more about the benefits of intermittent fasting and why it works so well for weight loss. If you're ready to jump in and just want to learn the different styles of fasting, skip to Chapter 7.

CHAPTER 3

How the Body Gets Energy While Fasting

Any day of the year, whether you're fasting or feasting, the body gets energy from either glucose or fat. Amino acids from proteins can also provide energy, but since protein is so vital to body functions, there are many mechanisms in place to spare amino acids from being used for energy (one of which is the production of ketones, as you shall see in this chapter). In a healthy person who eats a typical diet of carbs, fats, and proteins, the body will primarily use glucose for energy during and after meals, and primarily fat when it has been a long time since a meal. A metabolically healthy person will swing back and forth between functioning on a glucose-based metabolism and a fat-based one, a lot like a hybrid vehicle that can be alternately powered by electricity or gasoline, depending on its mode of operation.

The main signal that tells the body which fuel source to use is insulin. In a healthy person, when insulin levels are high, the main fuel source will be glucose. When insulin levels are low, fat will take over as the main energy source. If you follow a ketogenic diet, then you should have persistently low insulin levels and your "car" will mostly run on fat, without switching over to the glucose fuel. But remember: that fat can come from either foods you eat or the fat you carry on your body, depending on how much you're eating. So if it's weight loss that you're after, don't add too much new fat to the existing supply! Spend some time fasting, even if you are following a ketogenic diet.

Since the human body needs energy *all the time*, regardless of whether food is available, it developed very good mechanisms for storing energy after food is taken in and later drawing on those storage depots when food is not available. For most of human history, food was much more scarce than it is today, and the body needed to use these stores a lot. Because of this ability to store food energy, we don't have to eat all the time. There's no physical need for a regular daily meal schedule. The default pattern of breakfast, lunch, and dinner is just something we made up! You have no obligation to follow it.

Energy Storage

The body has specific storage depots for both glucose and fat. Glucose is only stored for short-term use, about a day or so. Fat storage, on the other hand, is apparently limitless. An average person can go some weeks without eating, relying exclusively on their body fat for energy. Someone with more fat can, as a general rule, fast longer than a thin person if they have the water, vitamins, and minerals they need.

Glucose Storage

Glucose comes into the body when you eat any carbohydrate food. All carbohydrates, not just things we think of as sweets or starches, are eventually broken down to release glucose into the bloodstream. Broccoli, sweet potatoes, spinach, rice, chocolate chips, nectarines, lettuce, you name it—they all contain carbohydrates that will convert to glucose for energy metabolism. The pancreas releases insulin, which helps direct glucose to three places:

1. to body cells, where it's used up for energy

2. to the liver and muscles for short-term storage, and

3. to be converted to fat and stored in fat cells for long-term use.

Glucose is stored in a chain called glycogen in the liver and muscles for the short term. A good amount of glycogen is stored in skeletal muscle for local use, but liver glycogen can supply energy for the rest of the body. You could think of liver glycogen like a candy necklace, where each little bead is one molecule of glucose and the necklace can only fit 100 beads. When there is a need for glucose, as is the case a few hours after a meal, the liver pops off those sugary little beads one at a time to feed into the bloodstream, where they can travel to cells that need them. The next time you eat carbohydrates, new beads of glucose are strung onto the chain until it's full again, with 100 beads. Later, when it's been a while since you've eaten, the process of releasing the beads into the bloodstream is repeated, and the necklace is left half full. When you eat another meal containing carbohydrates, your glycogen stores are replenished again. And so on.

If you don't eat (or don't eat carbs) and the body dips into your glycogen stores, they will only last about a day. The brain is a big energy hog, and it gobbles up much of the glucose the liver sends out from glycogen. After one day of fasting, when you have depleted your glycogen stores, the brain still wants to be fed, and the body will have to turn elsewhere for its glucose supply.

Glycogen and Water Weight

About 100 grams of glycogen are stored in the liver, and roughly 300 to 400 grams are stored in muscles (muscle glycogen stores vary depending on the person's size and body composition). Three grams of water are stored with each gram of glycogen. Therefore, the number you see on the scale will be a bit lower after you've depleted your glycogen stores after your first day of fasting.

Weight of total body glycogen:
100 grams liver glycogen
+ 300 grams muscle glycogen
= 400 grams (or 0.4 kilograms) body glycogen

Weight of water stored with glycogen:
400 grams body glycogen
× 3 grams water per gram of glycogen
= 1200 grams (1.2 kg) water

When you deplete your glycogen stores and the water stored with it, you lose 1.6 kg (0.4 kg of glycogen and 1.2 kilograms of water). One kilogram equals 2.2 pounds, so 1.6 kg × 2.2 = 3.5 pounds.

This is why people talk about losing a couple of pounds of "water weight" on the first day of their fast or on a ketogenic diet, and why, if they go back to eating carbs and refill their glycogen stores, they will gain those few pounds back right away. This is also one of the reasons why using a scale to measure success with fat loss is not optimal. Scales cannot tell you where the weight is stored! It's better to observe your waistline, how your clothes fit, and how toned your muscles are.

Fat Storage

The body can't store very much food energy as glucose. But we must store it somehow, so of course, it is stored as fat! When we talk about fat being stored in the body, we are really referring to triglycerides. You have probably heard this term before when you had blood work done at an annual physical. Fat is stored in a triglyceride molecule, which has two parts: fatty acids, or what we'll refer to as "fat" for simplicity's sake, and another part called glycerol, which is actually used to make glucose inside the body. It's worth repeating that *any* extra energy in the diet is stored as fat. So, if you eat too much carbohydrate, you won't store it as glucose—after you've filled your glycogen stores—you'll turn it into fat and store it as triglycerides in your fat cells. Fat stores in your body will continue to grow as long as you continue to feed them!

When triglycerides come out of storage to be used for energy, they are broken down into fatty acids and glycerol, which are used in separate pathways for energy production. Glycerol is used to produce glucose, while some fatty acids are used directly by cells and some are converted into ketone bodies in the liver. So in addition to storing a large quantity of energy, fat stores are really quite diverse and can supply energy via three different types of molecules that serve the body's needs in different ways, as you'll see in the following pages.

How long could that magnificent storage depot feed you if you suddenly found yourself alone on a desert island without food? To put things in perspective, if an average 145-pound person has a body fat percentage between 15 and 30 percent, they will have 10 to 20 kg of body fat on them, averaging 15 kg (15,000 g). Fat provides energy at a rate of 9 calories per gram, so 9 cal x 15,000 g = 135,000 cal. That's two months' worth of energy! Compare that to one day's worth of glucose in storage and you can easily see that the body is designed to meet its long-term energy needs using fat. Eighty percent of the body's energy is stored as fat. The table below compares glucose and fat stores in the body.

Indeed, there are reports of people fasting for two months or longer under medical supervision to reduce significant obesity (see page 105). But a prolonged fast is not something to take lightly. There is a tremendous difference between the simple practice of fasting for 24 hours on alternating days and the complicated matter of going without food for weeks or months, which can be deadly.

Fat versus Glucose Storage

Fuel source	Amount in typical 145-lb. person	Energy	Length of energy supply
Glycogen (glucose)	450 g	1800 cal	18 hours
Fat	15,000 g	135,000 cal	55 days

Different Cells Use Different Fuels

So far, we have seen that there are stores of glucose and fat in the body, but the amount of fat far exceeds that of glucose.

We know that over a long period of time without food, the body turns to fat for energy. But it's not quite as simple as that.

There are many different types of cells in the body, and they don't all have equal capacity to use fat or glucose as a fuel. Some cells are more flexible than others are. Cells in the heart, for instance, can use fat, ketones, and glucose. The cells in the brain and central nervous system prefer to use glucose, if it's available, or they can use ketones, but they can't use fat. Muscle cells can use fat, ketones, and glucose, depending on what's available and on what type of work the muscle is doing at the time.

So you can see that some cells are like the open-minded eaters in your group of friends—they'll have Italian, Mexican, Chinese, Thai, or anything else for dinner, depending on what's convenient. We want to convince more cells to be like these open-minded eaters and consider fat as a fuel source. That will help us achieve our goal of losing body fat.

The ability of your cells to use and easily switch between different fuels is called "metabolic flexibility." One of the goals of intermittent fasting is to improve metabolic flexibility. What affects metabolic flexibility? Some things you unfortunately can't change, like your genes, and how you've eaten and exercised all your life up to now. And some things you *can* change, like your level of fitness, your body composition, your stress and sleep levels, and how you choose to eat and exercise going forward. We'll talk more about how to improve your overall metabolic flexibility in Chapter 5.

The Body's Glucose Factory

Regardless of how metabolically flexible your system is, certain cells are not at all flexible when it comes to their energy source. These are like the picky eaters among your friends who always have to choose the restaurant and will take the whole group out of the way just to find the one thing they will eat. And this is where things start to get interesting when it comes to fat burning and ketosis.

Red blood cells, a part of the kidney called the renal medulla, certain cells in the eye, and some others can *only* use glucose for energy. And because we have no way to store glucose for long-term use (remember that the body has only about a day's worth of glycogen), we have to make our own glucose to feed these cells from the second day of fasting and beyond. Many people are surprised to find out that humans can make their own glucose! This flies in the face of the (bad) advice they have been getting that you have to eat carbohydrates every day to fuel the brain.

The process of making new glucose is called gluconeogenesis— *gluco* for glucose, *neo* for new, and *genesis* for creation. The ingredients for gluconeogenesis come from body fat, muscle tissue, and the recycled products of other metabolic processes. Only certain materials can be turned into glucose. Specifically, only the glycerol portion of a fat (triglyceride) molecule contributes to gluconeogenesis—the fatty acid portion gets used by cells that can use fat directly, or is converted to ketones for those that cannot. Certain amino acids, especially alanine and glutamine, are heavily relied upon to produce new glucose; these come from breakdown of muscle tissue and other means.

The body is very good at recycling nutrients. Muscle cells use the branched-chain amino acids valine, leucine, and isoleucine; conveniently, the process of breaking these down for energy releases alanine and glutamine, which are then diverted into glucose production. Lactate, released when muscle cells use glucose for energy while doing certain types of work (you may be familiar with lactic acid, which causes the "burn" with muscle exercise), is essentially a waste product that's recycled to create new glucose. The red blood cells and the renal medulla that are so dependent on glucose *also* produce lactate in the process of using it, and so provide some of the raw materials for the production of the very nutrient they need to survive in a continuous cycle of reuse.

So we have mechanisms to produce the glucose the body needs, even if no food is being consumed.

Glucose Is Not an Essential Nutrient

The name we give for nutrients that the body needs and cannot make, like vitamin C or magnesium, is "essential." You may know that certain amino acids are essential (leucine, lysine, methionine) and certain others are non-essential (alanine, glutamine) because we can make them inside the body from other materials. Similarly, linoleic acid (an omega-6 fat) and alpha-linolenic acid (an omega-3 fat) cannot be made in the body and must be consumed in the diet in order for a person to survive; therefore, these fatty acids are essential.

It's easy to believe that glucose—and therefore carbohydrates—is essential, because we know some cells need it. But since we can make glucose from other materials inside the body, using gluconeogenesis, it doesn't need to be consumed in the diet.

How long can this process of gluconeogenesis feed the cells and organs that require glucose? After two days of fasting, with glycogen stores long depleted, the brain, red blood cells, and renal medulla all still receive a constant supply of glucose from gluconeogenesis. The system can continue this way for another day or so.

But it can't keep going like that on such a limited glucose supply. Remember that we need some amino acids for gluconeogenesis. Some amount of muscle protein will be sacrificed to provide these amino acids. But muscle is important, and we don't want to lose too much. If the body's only long-term strategy for providing fuel for the brain were to sacrifice muscle mass to produce the needed glucose, then after a couple of days of fasting, we would become physically weak, distracted, and unable to concentrate. So what would have happened to our cavemen ancestors when, after a short famine, they came across an animal to hunt and eat? They would have been ill-equipped to chase down the potential meal and would have starved to death. Had that happened, you and I would not be here right now.

But of course, we are here, so we know that the caveman had a long-term strategy to meet the body's energy needs *without* sacrificing protein from his muscles.

Ketones Solve Two Big Problems

Humans can starve for a period of time without our muscle tissue wasting away because we can produce ketones, which can provide energy to the brain. Remember, the brain uses about a fifth of the body's energy, and it's metabolically "expensive" to provide that amount of energy in the form of glucose made in part from amino acids. You might think, "Hmm, if only the brain could use fat like all the other organs, that would really solve our problems." And that's where ketones come in.

Ketones are made from fat, and the brain can use them as an alternative to glucose. Hooray! We've got lots of fat. Producing ketones is a way to make fat do more jobs in the body and get used up more quickly. This adaptation helps conserve body protein during prolonged periods without food. It's one of the reasons why muscle mass is not rapidly lost during a fast to provide amino acids for glucose production. I've heard some people say that they are worried about being in ketosis because the body "catabolizes body protein," i.e., breaks down muscle to produce ketones. That's not true. Ketone production "catabolizes" (or breaks down) fat, if you want to phrase it that way, and actually helps protect against breakdown of body protein.

Ketones are always being produced, but in such small amounts that they are barely detectable in the blood stream and make no meaningful contribution to the body's energy needs. An extended period of low insulin levels and dwindling glycogen stores will increase production of ketones to physiologically significant levels, and a fast that extends beyond the point of glycogen depletion will boost ketone production further. Ketosis begins at a low level, for most people, after an overnight fast. Individual differences in biology determine how quickly, and to what degree, ketosis occurs after some hours or days of fasting.

We can also look at this adaptation as a way to spare glucose for the tissues that really need it. In the fasted state, skeletal muscle will shift almost entirely to fatty acids for its energy needs. The brain shifts to using ketones for two-thirds of its energy. But the red blood cells and the renal medulla still need glucose, and they can be fed now with the smaller supply that is available.

So now you have an idea of what is happening in ketosis, and why a period of two to three days or longer without food can promote significant fat loss without simultaneously promoting rapid loss of muscle mass.

Fuel Sources for the Brain during a Fast

	Eating day	Day 1 of fast	Day 2–3 of fast	Day 4 of fast and beyond
Main fuel for the brain	Glucose	Glucose	Glucose, ketones	Up to ⅔ of the brain's energy comes from ketones, and the rest from glucose
Primary fuel source	Meals	Glycogen, gluconeo-genesis	Gluconeogenesis, ketogenesis	Ketogenesis, gluconeogenesis

Ketone Testing

Ketones provide for less than 5 percent of the body's energy needs after an overnight fast, and about 30 to 40 percent of the body's energy needs after three days of fasting. As a fast progresses and more fat is burned for energy, the blood level of ketones rises. Consequently, many people are interested in testing their ketone levels to see how "deep into ketosis" they are and/or how fast they achieve ketosis.

There are three ketone bodies of interest: the first is aceto-acetate (AcAc), which gets converted into two other ketones, 3-β-hydroxybutyrate (3HB) and acetone. Of these, 3HB is the ketone that circulates in the blood stream and provides the majority of ketone energy to the body.

There are also three types of testing to measure the three types of ketones. Urine strips are by far the most common testing tool of the average ketogenic dieter. They're inexpensive, easy to get at any pharmacy, and don't require pricking oneself with a needle. Unfortunately, urine ketone measurement doesn't accurately reflect ketone use in the body. Urine strips measure acetoacetate that is spilling out in the urine. The body is getting rid of ketones it can't use by excreting them in the urine. This isn't the goal! The goal is to use ketones for cellular energy. When cells are well adapted to using ketones for energy, the body retains the acetoacetate rather than wasting it in the urine. So, urine strips will generally show "less ketosis" (i.e., less wasting of ketones through the urine) as the body's ability to use ketones increases. Therefore, urine strips are unable to give any meaningful result—a high reading means the body is wasting ketones (not ideal), and a low reading either means you're not producing ketones in sufficient quantity to measure (i.e., you're not in ketosis), or that your body has become quite good at using ketones and has stopped excreting them in the urine (i.e., you're keto-adapted). Urine strips aren't very useful as a measuring tool.

Breath ketone detection devices measure acetone, which is excreted through the breath. This is probably the second most common measurement tool among keto dieters. Although a breathalyzer is more expensive than urine strips, it's only a one-time purchase (about $75 to $150). And no needle pricking is required for this method, either. Unfortunately, there is disagreement over whether breath ketone meters can give a reliable sense of blood ketone levels, and consistency of results is considered poor.

Blood ketone measurements are the most accurate but least convenient testing method. For those who really want to understand how different foods or types of exercise impact their ketone levels, or simply how ketone levels change with fasting time, then blood ketone testing of 3HB levels is the way to go. Blood testing requires pricking your finger with a needle and dropping blood onto a testing strip. It's also more expensive than the other two methods—a blood ketone testing meter for at-home use can be purchased for as little about $50, but the testing strips are pricey and the cost adds up over time. But if you're really curious about your how your metabolism is affected by your fast or a ketogenic diet, then it may be worth the inconvenience! A good level of ketosis will correlate for most people with a BHB level of 1.5 to 3.0 mmol/L. You can measure your blood ketones upon waking, after each meal or snack, and before bed. You'll be able to see how different foods and activities impact your blood ketone levels and can use that information to fine-tune your diet or fasting window.

CHAPTER 4

Hunger and Satiety

Intermittent fasting gives you free reign to eat what and when you want as long as you're within your eating window. Still, it's worth embracing my number one rule for weight loss: if you're not hungry, don't eat. I don't care if it's dinner time. Your body doesn't seem to need food, so why feed it? Consider yourself lucky for the extra hour, and go do something else! Take a walk, call a friend, clean your house, organize your vacation photos—use the time for something other than adhering to a made-up meal schedule.

This urge to eat on a socially acceptable schedule is something we really buy into as adults. Children have a much better understanding of their physical need for food, and if you watch them, you'll notice they eat at irregular intervals, sometimes eating a lot, sometimes eating two bites or simply rejecting a meal outright (much to their parents' concern). Yes, they're growing, but that's not the only reason they eat that way. They are also better at responding to what they need and don't need when it comes to nourishment. Some very clever studies have shown that at the age of three, children are able to tell when they're full and stop eating, whereas by age six, children start to become as confused as adults about when to stop eating. They respond more to whether there is food in front of them than to whether they're hungry. They begin to eat more than they need, and they will probably do so for a lifetime.

But eating just because food is available or because it is a certain time of day is not the best strategy for weight loss. Feeling hungry sometimes is okay. No harm will come to you. But what makes us hungry anyway? Is there anything we can do to lessen sensations of hunger when we diet?

How Hunger Works

Many factors contribute to a feeling of hunger and the desire to eat or stop eating. Internally, hormones released in response to nutrients from a meal signal that the body has had enough nutrition, which prompts us to put down to the fork. A drop in nutrient availability (as happens when it's been a while since a meal, or after intense exercise) will turn up the appetite, as will certain hormones released in response to circadian rhythm or nutrient balance. Externally, the smell of food or the sight of an appealing dish can make us start salivating, signaling the beginnings of digestion and the body's anticipation of food to come. After you've eaten a lot, these same sights and smells might make you feel a little queasy, reminding you that fullness or satiety is just as real a sensation as hunger.

Ghrelin, the Hunger Hormone

One of the most powerful tools the body has to persuade you to eat is the hormone ghrelin. Ghrelin is often called the "hunger hormone" because it's produced by an empty stomach to tell the brain to increase appetite. It makes you eat more, and promotes fat storage. So you're probably not a fan of ghrelin!

But it makes sense that the body would have a mechanism to increase hunger when it senses that no food is coming in. The body is smart, and wants to prompt you to eat so it can store some food energy for future times of scarcity, when it'll have to get by on your fat stores. Of course, that's unlikely to happen in North America in the 21st century, but ghrelin doesn't know that.

One of the reasons some people are reluctant to try fasting is that they think they will just get hungrier and hungrier until they finally give in and eat. There's a misconception that ghrelin levels increase steadily the longer you go without food. But that's not how ghrelin works. Think about a time when you were hungry but engrossed in a project at work and just didn't have a chance to eat. Maybe the work distracted you from feeling hungry and you were surprised to notice a few hours later that your hunger was gone. That's how ghrelin works—it comes in waves. The timing of ghrelin release is affected by your typical meal schedule, which is one reason why you'll get hungry around the same time every day. It's also why, if you start skipping a given meal consistently, you're likely to be less hungry at that time of day. Hungry or not, it's helpful to know that ghrelin will make your stomach grumble and make you feel hungry, and then after a while the feeling will pass and you won't be hungry at all.

When you start fasting and you notice that sensation of hunger, you'll have to decide if you want to wait out the ghrelin peak, stick with the fast, and keep burning fat, or eat and suppress the sensation (food rapidly drives down ghrelin levels). If you wait it out, your hunger will later decrease and you'll be able to go a few more hours without eating or feeling hungry. That's the great thing about ghrelin peaks and dips—if you get through the peak, the dip will work in your favor. What's more, ghrelin has some positive effects in the body. It stimulates the release of growth hormone. Growth hormone, if you recall from Chapter 2, helps break down and get rid of body fat and build up muscle tissue. So if you can stick with your fast and ride one or two waves of a ghrelin peak, some very good things will happen!

If you choose to respond to ghrelin by eating, your fast will be broken, insulin levels will rise, and you won't start burning body fat again until a few hours after your meal. The option to eat is always available to you, though you often won't take it. Above all, be sure that you take good care of yourself and allow some flexibility in your fasting practice. Some days you'll be more interested in going longer before eating—or more likely, you'll just be busier and won't really notice the hunger, which is why one of the tricks to fasting successfully is to keep busy. Other days, you'll hear ghrelin shouting at you and you will choose to eat so that it quiets down. And that's perfectly fine. Fasting should be challenging and push you to be more flexible with your eating habits. But it should not be so uncomfortable that you're miserable. You're trying to develop a new habit that you can stick with for a lifetime—and no one would keep up with something that makes them miserable!

Getting Acquainted with Ghrelin

The more you practice fasting, the less bothered you'll be by ghrelin's chirping at you to eat something. There are a couple of other practical things to know about ghrelin activity when you're planning a fasting schedule.

1. Ghrelin levels tend to be lowest in the morning, around 8 to 9 a.m. So I'll say it again for good measure: if you're not hungry for breakfast, don't eat it!

2. Ghrelin levels peak and dip a couple of times a day. The peaks will correspond to your typical mealtimes,

and last about two hours. If you change your meal pattern, your hunger pattern is likely to change along with it.

3. For those who want to try fasts of more than a day, know that ghrelin levels are highest on day 2 of a fast and decrease steadily thereafter.

Leptin, a Satiety Hormone

The whole story of how the body receives hunger and satiety signals is complex, and better suited to an endocrinology textbook. So we'll just get acquainted with one more celebrity hormone before we move on.

You may have heard of the hormone leptin, secreted by fat cells, which sends signals to the brain about the size of the body's fat stores to help regulate appetite and energy expenditure. People with more fat have more leptin. If all is working as it should, an overweight person will secrete a lot of leptin, which will reduce their appetite and make their body use more energy, thereby reducing the size of their fat stores and restoring balance to the system. But things can go awry if a person has much too much fat and leptin. In that scenario, the brain becomes resistant to leptin's signals and the person doesn't get the message to eat less; as they continue to eat and store more fat, the fat cells produce more leptin, which just makes the whole problem worse. This is called leptin resistance, and it's similar to the problem of insulin resistance we discussed in Chapter 2. People who are leptin resistant won't get the benefit of a reduced appetite that leptin should provide, because the system is broken. Losing some body fat will reduce leptin levels and allow the brain to become re-sensitized to it.

Other Contributing Factors

Ghrelin isn't the only thing that makes us hungry, and leptin isn't the only thing that tells us to stop eating. There are many hormones that influence hunger and satiety, and other mechanisms in the body for regulating food intake. For instance, peptide YY is a hormone released from the small intestine in proportional response to food intake (more food, more peptide YY). It slows the movement of food through the digestive tract and binds to receptors in the brain that make you feel full. Like other hormones, it peaks and falls: levels are highest in the second hour after a meal and fall steadily thereafter.

In addition to hormones, there are other physiologic cues that adequate food has been eaten, or that more food is needed. For instance, certain sensors in the lining of the stomach stretch when food is eaten to signal the brain to decrease appetite. Foods and beverages that cause expansion of the stomach work through this mechanism to create satiety. This is one of the ways that fiber, which expands to absorb water in the digestive tract, helps to create a sense of fullness. Another trick sometimes used by people who fast is to drink lots of water to expand their belly if they want to prevent hunger. Deficiency or insufficiency of micronutrients can increase hunger and food intake. You can avoid this by eating a nutritious diet that provides adequate vitamins and minerals, or by taking a supplement to fill in any gaps if you feel your diet is falling short.

It's interesting to realize that even though the body has such sophisticated mechanisms for controlling food intake to match its energy needs, hunger levels go way down after a couple of days of fasting, when we would imagine nutrients are sorely needed. Ghrelin levels peak on day 2 of a fast and steadily decline thereafter, allowing hunger and the desire to eat to subside. Ketones, present in significantly higher amounts after two days of fasting, dampen the appetite as well. A conclusion can be drawn that a few days of fasting doesn't rob the body of nourishment that it needs, and that short periods of fasting are not harmful. If the body was starving, it would use all the tools it has—notably, ghrelin and the sensation of hunger—to make you uncomfortable and persuade you to eat. But the opposite is true: most people feel very well after a couple of days of fasting and don't really have a desire to eat.

It's Good to Skip Meals!

I hope I have convinced you by now that it's okay to skip meals. If you want to avoid gaining weight, it's a good idea not to eat when you're not hungry. If you're overweight, skipping meals when you're not hungry is a no-brainer. Skipping meals when you are hungry is a bit harder, but I imagine you've done much harder things in your life and I have no doubt you can do this too. If you can give yourself permission to set aside the hunger until it dissipates instead of reaching for a snack, and you can do that through breakfast and lunch twice a week, then you'll be intermittent fasting for 48 hours each week! That's 48 hours that you'll give your body to burn through your fat stores, helping you lose the extra weight you're carrying. That's a really good thing!

If I haven't convinced you by now that the body can thrive without three meals a day, I think I may know why. It's breakfast, isn't it? You have heard all your life that no matter what, you must not skip breakfast. Breakfast can be the last holdout. I hope you can believe me when I say that eating breakfast will not make you a healthier person. And moreover, eating before the hour of 9 a.m. does not magically make you lose weight. Eating breakfast is not the nutritional equivalent of doing three high-intensity interval workouts a week. It offers no special advantage to your metabolic health. It's just a meal eaten in the morning—and one that most Americans can't manage to consume without a day's worth of sugar. If you are actually hungry when you wake up in the morning, then go ahead and eat breakfast. Choose something high quality that's rich in protein and/or fat, with no sugar or flour. But if you are someone who does not get hungry in the morning, consider yourself lucky! You've been granted a free pass and can sidestep the nutritional landmine that is Breakfast in America. Please, for heaven's sake, skip it. Skipping breakfast will not do you harm.

Don't believe me? Then believe Mark Mattson. A 2016 article in *The New York Times* titled "Fasting Diets Are Gaining Acceptance" said this about Mark: "Mark Mattson, a neuroscientist at the National Institute on Aging in Maryland, has not had breakfast in 35 years. Most days he practices a form of fasting—skipping lunch, taking a midafternoon run, and then eating all of his daily calories (about 2,000) in a six-hour window starting in the afternoon." Mark Mattson has devoted his entire professional life to the study of healthy aging at the biggest health research organization in the country. If he thinks skipping breakfast is such a good idea that he's been doing it for 35 years, then maybe the rest of us should get on board.

CHAPTER 5

Metabolic Flexibility and Using More Energy

If your cells are not already well-equipped to use fat for fuel, then in order to take full advantage of the fat burning bene-fits of intermittent fasting, you need to help your cells become more metabolically flexible. We touched on this concept in Chapter 3.

Your body has many specialized cells, such as red blood cells, brain cells, and muscle cells, each of which need energy to do their cellular work. For example, liver cells work to detox-ify substances that come into the body and kidney cells work to filter the blood and create urine. Most of the energy your body uses in a given day powers these functions, which are the minimum processes needed to keep your body alive and well. The sum total of all the energy needed for these minimum required tasks is called Resting Energy Expenditure, or REE. This energy comes from the macronutrients—carbohydrates, fats, and to a lesser extent, protein or amino acids (though, as discussed previously, protein contributes relatively little to the body's energy needs because it is needed for other things).

What Is Metabolic Flexibility?

For the purpose of providing energy to cells, carbs are broken down into glucose, and fats are broken down into fatty acids (and later ketones). Fat and glucose are the major fuel sources, and many cells can make use of either depending on what's available and what is needed at the time. Muscle cells, for instance, want to use fats while at rest, and glucose when they're contracting, such as during exercise. In a healthy person, these cells will be able to shift back and forth between the fuels as the situation demands, and get energy from either one without difficulty. But this is not always the case. With poor eating and sleep habits and lack of exercise, the cells can become metabolically inflexible—meaning they can't use the different fuels very well, or switch back and forth between them. The classic case of this is someone with diabetes: they can't use glucose very well, so it remains in their bloodstream and promotes weight gain due to persistently high insulin levels.

What makes a healthy cell choose one fuel over another? It depends on a number of factors, including:

Availability. Are you fasting and have only fat as an energy source? Or did you just eat a high-carb meal and deliver a lot of glucose to your bloodstream?

Familiarity. Have you been eating only carb-heavy meals your whole life, and snacking constantly? Have you been on a ketogenic diet and/or intermittent fasting for a long while? This will impact the expression of genes and the concentration of compounds needed to metabolize glucose or fat.

Fitness of cells. What is the ability of your cells to extract energy from either fat or glucose? This is dependent in part on your overall fitness level, which is influenced by the type of exercise you do, as well as genetics.

It is essential to maintain your metabolic flexibility. Without it, you are much more likely to gain weight or have trouble losing it, suffer from lack of energy, and eventually develop diabetes. We want our cells to be able to easily use fats for energy when we are fasting, or when the muscles are at rest (e.g., sitting or sleeping). And we want the cells to be able to use glucose easily for energy when a meal delivers glucose to the bloodstream, or when the muscles are doing intense work (e.g., sprinting, lifting a heavy weight).

This concept is so important that I interviewed two experts on the subject to explain in their own words why metabolic flexibility is important, and how to maintain (or regain) your metabolic flexibility. The first interview is with J. Stanton, who studies nutrition and metabolism and who wrote the article "The Science Behind the Low-Carb Flu" in April 2011. He is among the first to introduce the concept of metabolic flexibility to the low-carb and ketogenic communities. The second interview is with Mike Nelson, a professor of exercise physiology, owner of Extreme Human Performance, and the creator of the Flex Diet Certification at flexdiet.com. Mike has a bachelor's degree in natural science, a master's in biomechanics, and a PhD in exercise physiology looking specifically at heart rate variability and metabolic flexibility.

Interview with J. Stanton

Subject: Metabolic Flexibility

Q: *Can you explain in one or two sentences what metabolic flexibility is?*

A: Metabolic flexibility is the ability of an individual cell to switch back and forth between fat and glucose as its energy source, based on the availability of these resources in our bloodstream. In healthy people, most cells in the body have this ability.

Q: *How does someone lose their metabolic flexibility?*

A: In simplified terms, metabolic flexibility is lost by a combination of excessive carbohydrate consumption and excessive omega-6 fatty acid consumption. Lack of exercise (both strength and endurance) and continual snacking likely accelerate the process.

Q: *What are the consequences of being metabolically inflexible? I mean, if my body is getting all the energy it needs, why does it matter what "fuel" I'm burning?*

A: Metabolic inflexibility means that, instead of switching back and forth depending on what's available, you're stuck burning a mixture of fat and glucose. This is bad for many reasons.

1. If we eat carbohydrates and sugars, and we can't switch to burning them, we can't dispose of them as quickly as we should. This causes poor glycemic control: high blood sugar spikes after meals, wide blood sugar swings and crashes, and the health and mood problems they cause.

2. When we fast, our ability to burn our own fat is diminished, and we have a continual demand for carbohydrates, even at rest. This means we become hungry sooner after eating, and

become dependent on sugary, bready snacks to "keep our energy up."

3. If we manage to ignore these through willpower, and we diet or fast anyway, our bodies will reduce our metabolic rate, we will become tired and listless as well as hungry, and our diet will be very likely to fail.

Q: *How does someone regain metabolic flexibility?*

A: Metabolic flexibility toward glucose—the ability to use glucose efficiently for energy when appropriate—is regained by consuming less glucose (whether as sugars or as starches) than your body uses.

Metabolic flexibility toward fat—the ability to use fat efficiently for energy when appropriate—is regained by exercise. Fasting and dieting support the process, but are insufficient by themselves, because only exercise causes cells to rebuild their mitochondrial population. [Mitochondria are the specialized structures inside cells where fatty acids are broken down for energy. When we talk about "fat-burning machinery," we are referring in large part to mitochondria.]

Exercise causes your cells to build more mitochondria, and fasting—particularly fasted exercise—causes your cells to break down and recycle the least functional mitochondria and build new ones. Therefore, a combination of fasted and fed exercise will recycle and rebuild your mitochondria, and thus restore your ability to burn fat, to the extent this is possible for you. As I said before, "You can't exercise your way out of a bad diet—and you can't diet your way out of not exercising."

Q: *What are some specific ways that someone can put the above information to use right away?*

A: Take a brisk walk every morning, before you eat, and don't eat afterward until you're hungry. Don't jog, and stay off the treadmill and Stairmaster unless it's raining and you can't take a walk. Keep hard-boiled eggs around to snack on. If you're not hungry enough to eat a hard-boiled egg, you're probably not hungry, just bored. If you keep needing to snack between meals, you probably didn't eat enough, or you've been slacking off on your exercise.

Lifting heavy weights increases muscle mass, and therefore increases your body's ability to dispose of glucose, and calories in general. Once a week is enough to maintain general health, though you can lift more often if you really want to bulk up or lean out. Stay away from gimmicks: focus on basic compound movements like squats, pull-ups, rows, presses, and loaded carries. Everything else, from yoga to resistance bands, is a less-important and optional adjunct to basic strength training. (Note to women: you won't accidentally grow huge muscles if you start lifting! Instead, you will find is that it's much easier to maintain fat loss.)

Q: *What are your thoughts on intermittent fasting?*

A: If you're metabolically flexible and have no problems fasting, there's an argument for the deep autophagy produced by a multi-day fast. But, in my opinion, it's much easier to exercise while fasted and burn multiple days' worth of calories in a day than it is to sit around cold and tired for several days.

Since exercise restores mitochondrial function, which restores the ability to oxidize fat, I recommend that you start your exercise program before starting your intermittent fasting regimen.

In my readers' experience with intermittent fasting, men often do better by simply skipping breakfast and waiting until lunch to eat, while women often find greater success by eating a late breakfast and fasting until dinner. If one plan doesn't work, try the other.

Q: *How can readers find out more?*

A: They can reference the index to my articles on nutrition, metabolism, human evolution, and My Ancestral Health Symposium (AHS) 2013 presentation, "What Is Metabolic Flexibility, and Why Is It Important?" at www.gnolls.org/index.

Interview with Mike T. Nelson

Subject: Metabolic Flexibility

Q: *Can you explain metabolic flexibility to those of us who don't have a PhD in exercise physiology?*

A: Metabolic flexibility is how well your body can use the two main fuels, which are carbs and fats, and then how well you can switch back and forth between those two fuels.

Q: *How does someone lose their metabolic flexibility?*

A: Lots of things contribute: sedentary lifestyle, lack of exercise, caloric surplus. Pretty much any type of overeating will destroy metabolic flexibility; it doesn't matter what nutrient is being overconsumed. Sleep is important, too— just one night of missed sleep increases insulin resistance measurably. And stress: if you have more stress that you can handle, that can also do it.

Q: *What are the consequences of being metabolically inflexible?*

A: There may be some implications for athletic performance, and mostly an impact on metabolic health. I believe that if you're using high-intensity fuel like carbs all the time, even at rest, it's not the best for your metabolic health. You're not able to downshift to use fat for low-intensity exercise; you're just using glucose all day. If I'm a human and I'm hanging out watching TV, I should probably use the correct fuel for just hanging out and doing very little, which is fat.

Q: *How does someone regain their metabolic flexibility?*

A: The hard part about metabolic flexibility is there are two ends of the spectrum. People say, "I'm doing a ketogenic diet because I want to be more metabolically flexible." That's great if you want to use more fat and ketones. But if you stay in that metabolic state a long time, you'll lose the ability to use carbs. You're actually giving up some of that flexibility on the carb end of the spectrum. If you are looking to be better at using carbs for power or speed but have been on a high-fat, low-carb diet for some time, add in more carbs after a workout since your body can use glucose better after exercise.

Q: *How can you test metabolically flexibility without going to a lab?*

A: Have some carbs in isolation and then see how you feel. If you have a bowl of oatmeal and then you feel like you have to take a nap, then you're not so good at using carbs! Honestly, you should be able to have two pop tarts for breakfast and be okay. I'm not saying to do that every day—just as a test! On the other hand, can you go 12, 16, 24 hours without eating and also be okay? Then you know you're able to use fat well. It doesn't mean you need to fast every day; it's just a way to test your ability to use fat.

Q: *What are some specific ways that someone can put this information to use right away?*

A: Doing some type of fast for a period of time is a useful way to increase metabolic flexibility. I prefer fasting over a ketogenic diet because in the long term, on a ketogenic diet, you will start losing flexibility on the high-end carb metabolism side. With fasting, it appears you do not. So you could fast for 24 hours on Monday, get all the benefits of being in a ketogenic state, such as low insulin and maybe autophagy, and the next day go back to eating a moderate-carb diet, and you should be fine.

Also, make sure to include more movement in your life. It doesn't have to be formal exercise—just get a dog, take up a new sport, and move! If you can exercise, weight training has tons of benefits for metabolic health.

Using More Energy

In addition to making sure cells can easily use the energy you give them from fat or glucose, you also want to take steps to increase the amount of energy you use overall—i.e., your energy expenditure. Remember, extra energy from food you eat is stored as fat. The more energy you use, the less you will carry around with you. So how can you use more energy?

An important concern for someone on a weight loss diet is that it will slow down their metabolism, which over time will cause them to plateau and regain the weight. This is hugely important and should not be overlooked! We know that we not only want to lose weight, but also want to keep it off. One of the benefits of fasting for weight loss or maintenance is that fasting prompts release of the hormone adrenaline, which increases the metabolic rate. This is in contrast to a calorie-restricted diet, which tends to decrease the metabolic rate.

What do people actually mean when they say that dieting slows your metabolism or decreases your metabolic rate? They are really talking about the body's ability to reduce the amount of energy it uses in a given day, i.e., Total Daily

Energy Expenditure (TDEE). The amount of energy the body spends in a day is dependent on a number of factors, including: age, gender, the type and amount of food you eat, and the amount of muscle mass you carry on your body. It's also dependent on how much you move around, irrespective of how much "formal exercise" (e.g., hours on the elliptical machine) you do. Movement itself is key to using more energy.

Many people know that muscle mass uses more energy than fat mass, regardless of exercise regimen. Of course, it's exercise that maintains muscle mass in the first place! And some people worry about losing muscle when they diet. We have already seen that growth hormone triggered by intermittent fasting helps build muscle mass. It's also worth noting that we don't have to sit around and "worry" about losing muscle when we lose weight—we can actually get up and grow some more! Muscles get bigger when your body is convinced it needs bigger muscles to do more work. So, lift some heavy things, start including strength training in your exercise plan, and grow some bigger muscles!

Interview with Mike T. Nelson

Subject: Using More Energy

Q: *What is resting metabolic rate (RMR) or basal metabolic rate (BMR)?*

A: RMR is the amount of energy your body has to burn to just stay alive. If you're lying down watching TV, you're actually doing too much work to measure RMR. You have to be in the lab lying down with your eyes closed, doing nothing.

Q: *People on weight loss plans are often concerned about slowing their metabolism. True or false: resting metabolic rate can go up or down.*

A: Can your RMR change over time? Yes. Does it change as much as people think it does? No. It doesn't move that much.

What people are most interested in is REE, or resting energy expenditure. This includes RMR, NEAT (non-exercise activity thermogenesis), formal exercise, and the thermogenic effect of food (which is the cost to digest energy). RMR uses the most energy—around 50 percent. The one that's most controllable is your NEAT—how much you move, *aside from* formal exercise. A lot of your daily movement is unconscious (like shaking your leg, for instance), and that contributes to NEAT and daily energy expenditure.

So when people are thinking about slowing metabolism, it's mostly about total daily energy expenditure—which includes NEAT—and not so much RMR, which really doesn't change that much. RMR is how many calories it takes to keep you alive, and the main thing that changes it is lean body mass— the more lean body mass you have, the more energy you burn. But the changes are not very dramatic. Does increasing lean body mass increase RMR? Yes. Should you be doing things to bump up your lean mass over time? Yes. But is that the thing on a day-to-day basis that will have the biggest impact on overall metabolic rate? Nope. It's how much energy you're burning as you move around. It's NEAT.

Let's say you're eating 3000 calories a day, and then you slash your calories to 1500 per day because you're trying to lose weight on a low-calorie diet. Your RMR is not going to crash very much from that. What will go in the tank fast is your NEAT—how much you move around—and you won't even notice it! Your brain goes whoa, we better not move around very much because we don't have any calories coming in, so we can't afford to burn much energy. You start feeling lethargic, and you reduce unconscious movement. The formal exercise might not stop, because you may force yourself to go to the gym—but if you measure how many steps you take, and how much you fidget and just how much movement you have outside of exercise, it's much, much less. This is one of the major ways that low-calorie diets without variation in energy intake, over time, tend to reduce your daily energy expenditure and slow your metabolic rate.

Q: *What are some takeaways for people who want to increase their metabolic rate, or at least prevent weight loss from slowing their metabolism?*

A: It comes down to how many calories you burn per day, including how much you move around, which is in your control. It doesn't need to be "formal" exercise. Just get up, move around, go for a walk, do some yard work—anything but sitting around like a slug.

Doing some sort of weight training will expend more energy. Weight training does help prevent the drop in RMR. It doesn't lead to a big change, but it helps in the long term, since we know people are going to lose muscle over time. Keeping as much skeletal muscle as possible is a key component in the battle against future weight gain. And I think moderate-intensity exercise is great for aerobic development. I like this template: lift something Mondays, Wednesdays, and Fridays, and do some cardio Tuesdays, Thursdays, and Saturdays. If they can only do four days, dedicate two to lifting and two to cardio.

Protein has a higher thermic effect of food, which is another way the body uses energy—though it doesn't add up to a lot. Perhaps more important is that protein is extremely satiating for the amount of calories, so people are unlikely to eat a chocolate cake after they eat a good amount of protein. My recommendation for protein is 0.7 grams per pound of lean body mass.

Q: *Can you share some final thoughts on intermittent fasting?*

A: When I first heard about intermittent fasting about nine years ago, I thought it was a horrible idea. I tried it and I made it like 10 hours, and then I destroyed a Chinese buffet. But then I realized it was too much of a jump to go from my normal diet to a 24-hour fast, so I started pushing up breakfast every Monday by two hours. Then I started using it with clients and I found that most people could do one day of fasting much easier than one day of low caloric intake. If I told them not to eat for a day or gave them a chance to have 500 calories for lunch, the lunch thing didn't really work. Also, the rules are so easy: just don't eat anything with calories in it. People get it.

From a metabolic standpoint, there is a benefit to lowering insulin levels. Their insulin levels will flatline with a fast. High levels of insulin use carbs; with low levels of insulin, you use fat. It's like a metabolic switch. When you drop insulin, you get them to use fat. I'd love to see a study where people fast one day a week and see what fuels they're using—especially take a look at the people who, at baseline, are using glucose at rest (which is not ideal), and see them start to use fat at rest (which is ideal) when they're fasting, and then maybe even see them shift over to using fat at rest on the days they're not fasting, which is great. The body will almost always adapt to whatever you're doing, that's the beautiful thing.

Keep Your Metabolic Rate High: Get Moving

Maybe you know that movement is important to maintaining weight loss, but you don't have an exercise routine or you have struggled to start one. A lot of people are in your shoes, and there are smart ways to get started and keep going. I believe there are two main barriers that keep people from getting enough movement or exercise: The first is perceived lack of time, and the second is that they haven't found any activities they really enjoy.

Finding Time to Exercise

Whenever I start working with someone who tells me they don't exercise or just barely do so because they are just too busy, I have them do a couple of things to assess how they spend and perceive their time. I ask what percentage of their time they realistically feel they can devote to exercise now that weight loss is a priority for them. Most people tell me around 10 percent. To which I usually raise my eyebrows and say, "Wow! You're going to start doing 17 hours of exercise per week? That is really a lot!"

There are 168 hours in a week. Ten percent works out to 16.8 hours—way too much time to spend doing formal exercise. So I ask the busy people who are starting with zero hours of exercise per week to be a little more modest, and devote just 1 percent of their time to physical activity. That's 1.68 hours, or one hour and 45 minutes per week. This really puts in perspective how little you need to do to make an impact on your health and weight loss. Even the busiest of people find a way to do that.

If this sounds like you, take a piece of paper and track how you spend all 168 hours one week. List the days of the week at the top, and the activities—sleep, work, commuting, house chores, TV watching, time with family—on the side. Then just spend 2 minutes at the end of the day jotting down the number of hours you spend in each activity. After one week, many people find they've spent a dozen hours doing unimportant things. They come back and tell me they can easily double their exercise time to three hours per week. This person will spend one less hour on housework and two hours less watching TV, and they'll have three hours to exercise. By session two, we nip the "no time to exercise" problem in the bud!

Another interesting discovery on these time logs is the number of hours people spend preparing and consuming food. One of the great benefits of intermittent fasting, as I've mentioned before, is the enormous amount of time you'll save! If you currently cook your meals, you know it takes many hours every week to go to the grocery store, prep, cook, and of course, eat. Going out to dinner can be a two-hour affair. When you fast, you cut out multiple meals from your week and save a ton of time.

If you're someone who can't find the time to exercise, I recommend you try doing a weekly time log. It may be eye opening! If you haven't yet started your fasting schedule, consider doing a baseline time log and another a month or two after you've gotten into your fasting schedule—you may see significant time savings in the "food prep and eating" column.

Finding "Exercise" That You Enjoy

Not surprisingly, not everyone loves lifting weights or spending an hour on the elliptical machine. But you may think you're supposed to exercise this way, because those are the things that are readily available to most of us though fitness gyms.

As you've learned from the experts interviewed in this chapter, cardio machines are not the optimal path to weight loss and metabolic health! The best way to build muscles, prevent weight gain, and maintain your metabolic health is through regular movement of varying kinds. It does not have to be unappealing or excruciatingly difficult. It certainly *should not* be those things, or else you won't do it! It's best to find ways to move more in your daily life. Sprint to the bus stop, lift heavy rocks to clean up your backyard, play a round of basketball at the local park, dance to the tune of your favorite song, walk or bike anywhere you need to go—just get up and get moving while doing something that matters to you. Then, you are very likely to keep doing it.

A few years ago, I came across a study that made this point quite nicely. The study separated participants into two groups, gave all participants books to read, and tracked how often everyone went to the gym. The only difference between the groups was that the participants in one group had to leave their books at the gym and could only read while they were there, whereas participants in the other group could take their books home with them to read whenever they wanted. Who do you think went to the gym more? You guessed it: the people who left their books at the gym. They were willing to exercise more often in order to find out how the story would unfold! This drives home the point that attaching movement to something else that's important to you will increase the likelihood that you'll do it.

One of the best examples I've seen of this is when a married person who wants to spend more time exercising convinces their spouse to take a brisk nightly walk as part of their quality time together. Sometimes this is instead of or in addition to spending evening time on the couch in front of the TV. The benefit to the couple is that they both get healthy movement in their day, *and* they get quality time to talk and connect during their walk. It also eliminates the problem of deciding whether the gym is more important than time with your spouse! Some people make similar changes to interact in a physically active way with their children. They're motivated by the idea of quality time with those they love, so they play catch with the kids in the yard, or have a family run with the dog.

Other things may motivate you. If you want to make new friends, maybe an exercise class or yoga class is right for you. You might find a sports team you can join. If you like to contribute to a good cause, then you can easily find a charity that has training teams in your area for an annual fundraising event— for instance, you can train for a 5k to raise money for breast cancer research. Or volunteer to do something that requires movement instead of sitting still. I once volunteered for a day with Habitat for Humanity, an organization that builds houses for people in need of them. I was assigned to paint doors. Others were putting together house frames, and I thought I was getting off easy. Boy was I wrong! After a day of painting doors, my shoulders and biceps were so sore, I felt like I had done hours of weight lifting in the gym. But I dislike lifting weights, and I never would have done that much work in a gym environment. The experience of being with others contributing to a good cause was much more motivating to me, and I was happy to do it!

If you enjoy being in the outdoors, start doing activities outside. Hiking, biking, find a workout class in the park. Are there trails near your home that you've always wanted to explore? Grab a friend and take a bike or hike. Find a hill or inclined street in your neighborhood that looks like it would be a challenge to climb, and walk that direction. Do you find yourself driving to pick up your kids at a friend's home five minutes away? Walk there instead, and walk home with your kids so they can see a model of daily movement and grow up to value that in their own lives.

CHAPTER 6

How to Get Started If You're Unsure

If you have never tried to fast for any amount of time and can't imagine even skipping a meal—let alone a whole day of eating—then I invite you to take a deep breath and remember that you don't have to jump in with both feet. There are dozens of relatively easy things you can do to lower the psychological barrier to fasting. That's what this chapter is all about. Of course, if you're a "dive right in" kind of person and want to get going, then by all means, get to it! There is no special preparation needed to begin fasting. You can start now.

Group your eating moments—don't graze. First and foremost, distinguish mealtimes from all other times. You can eat any amount of food you want—just eat it at either breakfast, lunch, or dinner. Respect that all other times are non-eating times. If you want dessert after dinner, eat it in the same "eating moment" as dinner itself. Don't get up, clear the table, wash the dishes, retire to the couch for a movie, and *then* eat dessert.

Similarly, don't nibble before breakfast, or have a mid-morning snack after breakfast. If you are hungry before and after breakfast, make yourself a bigger breakfast. And if you normally have a snack a couple hours after lunch, add that snack to the end of your lunch. Then, wait to eat again until dinner.

Swap heavy cream for sugar in your coffee or tea, or take it plain. This is a small but significant move. Many of us drink coffee or tea once or more per day. The beverages themselves have great health benefits, and I generally don't see reason to restrict them. The trouble comes when you add sugar or other sweeteners to these beverages. They become just another source of sugar in our daily diets, and continue to reinforce the sugar cravings you are trying to put to rest. Instead of sugar, learn to take your coffee black and your tea plain. If you can't take it black, add heavy cream (not milk) or coconut oil or cinnamon if you like those flavors. Don't add almond milk or similar products that have carbohydrates, alternative sweeteners, or both. If you are fasting and want to take coffee or tea on your fasting day, it's helpful to get this practice under your belt.

Create a "no eating" buffer around your sleep time. If you're doing well with three meals a day and you aren't grazing or snacking in between, the next step is to create a mini "no eating" window after dinner and before breakfast. If you think about it, sleep is the longest period of fasting that most of us have every day—a nice eight hours or so. If you can push your first morning bite out two hours into the day, and make sure dinner wraps up two hours before bedtime, then you'll increase that fasting window by 50 percent! That's a fast of 12 hours, and is a real accomplishment. If this works for you, keep going that way, maybe pushing breakfast out two more hours the following week. You'll see that you may get to a 16-hour fast in no time.

Ask others about their fasting experiences. Fear of the unknown is one of the biggest challenges when it comes to fasting. For most of us who were raised in Western society, fasting is just not part of our culture. Its unfamiliarity makes it that much more intimidating.

So, don't venture into the great unknown all by yourself! Ask around your circles and find out who has a fasting practice, whether for weight loss, health, religious, or other reasons. They will have great advice to offer, and will be able to allay some of your fears. Join the *Delay, Don't Deny* Facebook group and start meeting people who practice fasting as a lifestyle. There are hundreds of groups and support circles out there. I am confident that you will find people in your social spheres who practice fasting, too. Personally, when I was looking to interview people about their fasting practices for this book, I simply asked around. I was surprised to learn that quite a few of my colleagues have a fasting practice, as well as a cousin of mine, and even some friends who work in the restaurant industry (not usually a place you find people turning down food!). So go find support to get started, and stay involved for the motivation to continue. There's nothing that helps a new habit stick better than being around others who practice the same.

Find a friend or family member who wants to try intermittent fasting with you. If you're not interested in asking far and wide and would rather have support closer to home, convince a family member or friend to try out a fasting practice with you. Preferably someone you share meals with, so you can organize the fast around your meal schedule and either do something else together during mealtimes, or break your fast together if the time is right. Maybe your spouse or partner is willing to do it, and you can both skip eating throughout the day, then come home to share a nice dinner together. Or maybe you have a coworker who wants to skip breakfast and lunch with you, and the two of you can take a quick walk on your lunch break instead of eating with the rest of the staff.

Finding a fasting partner not only creates accountability (you'll worry about letting them down if you "cheat"), but also a sense of companionship, someone to troubleshoot with and with whom to marvel at how easy it is after all. You'll feel you're not alone in the experience, that you have someone to call on who "gets it." In some ways, the gratification of sharing the experience may even be one of the things that motivates you to keep doing it.

Stop eating before your workout because you think you need the energy. Quit having a snack or energy drink or smoothie before a workout. If you exercise in the morning, experiment with a fasted workout. Make sure to drink water. You are likely to be just fine. If you're tentative about skipping the pre-workout snack, just take it a little slower than usual. The worst that could happen is you don't feel great afterward, so you take it easy and eat a meal and recover. But more likely, you will feel okay to try it again the next day.

That said, please use common sense: If you are very out of shape, haven't exercised in a year, and have never gone a few hours without eating in your entire life, don't just jump in and do a big workout in the middle of your first fast! That's when you are likely to feel unwell. If you're just starting to exercise *and* starting to work your fasting muscle, set off by doing 10 minutes of exercise in the fasted state, and if that goes well, up it to 20. Be mindful of your own limits.

Stop saying "I have to eat." One thing that fasting teaches is that eating is a choice. For many of us, we were raised with people saying how much we "have to" eat at the dinner table. Society tells us we "have to" eat three meals a day, or a friend tells us we "have to" eat if it's been some number of hours since our last meal. Ever wonder how they know when *your* body needs food? Or how about being told you "have to" eat when you're sick and can't stomach any food? Presumably this is to "keep up your energy" while you're fighting off the illness. Has it ever occurred to these advice-givers that the energy required to metabolize your meal might indeed be better spent fighting off that very illness?

People don't need food for all these arbitrary reasons. Once you get out of the habit of feeding the body simply to ease your emotional distress or the inflated concerns of those around you, then you will begin to see that the "have to eat" moments are really few and far between. Most of the time you are simply *choosing* to eat to avoid an uncomfortable situation. It's certainly your right to make that choice. Just know it's a choice, not a necessity. And perhaps start saying to yourself, "I'll eat now because it feels right for this situation, but I don't actually have to." Over time, if you're not achieving the results you want, you may decide that it's not worth it.

Give your meal your full attention. Since you will have distinct mealtimes and won't be mindlessly nibbling throughout the day, devote your full attention to your meal when you have one. And now that you've stopped believing eating is something you "have to" do at any given time, you may feel more empowered when making the choice to devote some of your precious time to eating. Revel in your own authority. Mark the transition from whatever else you're doing to the occasion of eating a meal. Don't drive, read, or work at the computer while you're eating. If you have only 10 minutes, take the 10 minutes to stop whatever else you're doing and just eat. Sit down to your meal without distraction. You will appreciate the experience more, and you will begin to approach food will more consideration.

Cut way down on sugar. You may notice that eating sugar causes your appetite to swing wildly, which can make it more difficult to go from one meal to the next without snacking. Since we want to avoid snacking, sugar is not on our side. It also undermines the great progress you make when you stop believing you have to eat and become the master of your own eating habits instead. I am generally pessimistic about someone's prospects for significant weight loss and weight maintenance if they have an attachment to sugary foods. Things like soda, juice, sweetened drinks, cookies, candies, cakes, ice cream, "food bars," muffins, chocolate-covered things, pastries, sweetened crackers, dessert tarts made with coconut sugar and other "healthy sweeteners," dried fruit—the list never ends. Intermittent fasting can be quite difficult if you eat these foods on a regular basis. Long-term health outcomes are likely to be poor. Sugar in the amounts we consume it is flat-out dangerous. It's best to cut it way down, or cut it out.

The good news is, sugar cravings go away rather quickly when you stop feeding them. I generally ask clients who want to stop eating sugar to commit to seven days with no sweets at all, and a reassessment at that time to decide if they want to extend their sugar fast. The first week is usually the hardest, so by day 7, it hardly seems worth throwing away all that good work, and they recommit to seven more days. If sweets have a hold on you, I recommend trying seven days of no sweets or, if that seems unrealistic, try seven days during which you'll only eat something sweet once per day. After that, you can pick a few days to have a sweet thing, and a few days to skip it. You can decide where you want to go from there. Life without attachment to sugar is better. It's a lot like life after quitting smoking. I've never heard anyone say they wish they still smoked. Ask someone who's kicked their sugar habit to tell you about it, and see for yourself.

Start eating more fat. Fat makes meals more satisfying so you can go longer between meals. Skip anything labeled "low-fat." Instead, use full-fat dressings on salads and eat full-fat cheese or yogurt. Add sliced avocado to any dish. Use tahini (a sauce made from sesame seeds) as a dip or sauce for vegetables. Eat a handful of nuts with a meal that isn't very high in fat to begin with. If you eat breakfast and enjoy eggs, always have the yolk (don't just eat the whites), and have bacon on the side. Cook vegetables in a good amount of coconut oil or olive oil. If you take cream in your coffee, make sure it's heavy cream and not milk. Experiment with fat coffee or "bulletproof" coffee: blend 1 or 2 cups of black coffee with 1 tablespoon of butter and 1 tablespoon of coconut oil for a frothy, creamy mixture to drink in place of a meal. It's quite filling and energizing.

Observe your current eating patterns to see where you can easily stick in a fast. Take a few days to pay close attention to *when* you eat. What's the first thing you put in your mouth after you wake up? Is it coffee or tea, breakfast food, or water? Or do you busy yourself getting ready for work and run out the door, grabbing a breakfast sandwich on the way? Maybe you eat nothing at all in the morning. Whatever it is, just take note of your pattern.

Do the same for moments later in the day. When do you eat lunch, or do you skip it on busy days? What are your snacking habits? Is dinner a family affair that happens around the same time every night, or is your schedule more irregular, with late dinners on some evenings and early ones on others? You may discover that you already go long periods without eating, and that a bout of intermittent fasting here and there would not be a huge change from your normal routine. Many people tell me they don't eat breakfast anyway and usually eat lunch around noon. It's within reach for them to stop putting sugar in their morning coffee (this is probably harder than not eating, actually, but you can do it in a week—see page 77), and quit snacking after dinner the night before, so they can achieve a

16-hour daily fasting window. Some people say that a certain day of the week is just chaos for them, and eating is impossible anyway. Do you have any days like this? Grab that opportunity!

Observe your hunger patterns. While you're observing your eating patterns, take careful stock of when you are hungry. Start by asking yourself if you're hungry in the moments before eating something, and note how soon after a meal or snack you are hungry again. Is the feeling of hunger what prompts you to seek out food? Or do you simply choose to eat at standard mealtimes or when food is around, regardless of whether you are hungry? I recommend you use a piece of paper or the notepad on your phone to make a list of your eating moments during the day, and note "yes" or "no" to the question of whether you were hungry before eating. It might look something like the chart below.

Eating versus Hunger Habits

Coffee and muffin on the way to work	Not sure I was hungry, but it's my morning routine
Salad at the lunch spot	Hungry
Mixed nuts at my desk	Not hungry
Dinner	Hungry
Ice cream	Not hungry, just wanted a treat

One of the biggest challenges to starting a fasting practice is the fear of being hungry. It might surprise you to learn that you're not always hungry when you reach for food—and perhaps this will give you the confidence to try and skip a meal without fear.

Set clear goals. Why are you interested in fasting in the first place? What exactly do you want to achieve? Be specific. "Lose weight" or "be healthy" are not specific goals. You want to set goals that are clear and easy to measure. I am not a fan of scales, because they can't tell you what portion of your weight is fat and what portion is lean mass. I find that how your clothes fit is a much better gauge of success with fat loss. So take some time to write or think about why you are doing this. Envision your success. You might say: "In six months with intermittent fasting, doing a 24-hour fast two times a week, I will fit into those pants." (You know which pants.) If at three months you are not halfway to your goal, you can adjust.

It also helps to find role models for success. Whom do you know who has done what you want to do? What does their success look like? Decide what you want, envision your success, and go after it.

If you're not sure how to get started, then *just start*. It's pretty easy to get started. If you are someone who eats three meals a day like clockwork, then start by skipping breakfast tomorrow, and the day after that. If you just ate lunch and feel very full, skip dinner tonight. If you are super motivated right now and want to get started with a 24-hour fast, don't eat again until lunch tomorrow. You really can start now. No time like the present.

CHAPTER 7

How to Practice Intermittent Fasting

When someone first starts fasting, they usually have a few questions: "Exactly how many hours it will take to get into ketosis?" "What level of ketosis should I aim for?" "How long do I have to fast for maximum fat burning?" These are all reasonable questions, but difficult to answer in a general sense. Many things influence the rate of ketone production; for instance, the amount of liver glycogen you had going into your fast (which is affected by how much carbohydrate you ate prior to fasting). If you typically eat a low-carb or ketogenic diet, then you won't lay down much glycogen at all and you'll enter a ketogenic state more quickly. The amount of exercise you do while you're fasting has an impact as well. This is pretty obvious, though—the more energy you use in the fasted state, the more fat and ketones will be used because those are your main energy sources during a fast. Your size and body composition matters, too, as well as how fit your muscles are and how good they are at using fats, glucose, and ketones.

So the focus on level of ketosis and exact timing to optimize ketone production is a bit misplaced. What's essential is that you keep up a fasting practice *and* have a varied exercise practice. Do that, and you will get better at producing and using ketones, and better at using fat directly, too. This is what you want.

It's also hard to tell exactly at what time of day your ketones levels will be highest. If you're looking for some marker to decide how long to fast, pay attention to how you feel. Fasting and ketosis increase your sense of well-being. They make you feel good. The caveat is you have to get through the transition from eating all the time and operating solely on a glucose-based metabolism, to eating less often and training your cells to use fat again. That's why I recommend a minimum six-week commitment to any fasting plan you start.

For the rest of this chapter, I'm going to outline some of the popular intermittent fasting patterns out there, simply because I think it helps to have some models when you're starting out. This chapter will also include interviews with people who incorporate intermittent fasting into their own lives, so you can see first-hand accounts of how it works. Remember, don't get too caught up in the precise timing or structure of these patterns. The important thing is to begin a fasting practice that is feasible for you and make it a consistent part of your life. There is no perfect schedule except the one that works for you.

Common Intermittent Fasting Schedules

	Time-restricted eating	5:2	Alternate-day fasting	Time-restricted eating plus a 24 hour fast
Mon	Eat only from 12 p.m.–8 p.m.	Eat normally	Eat normally	Eat only from 12 p.m.–8 p.m.
Tue	Eat only from 12 p.m.–8 p.m.	24-hour fast	24-hour fast	Eat only from 12 p.m.–8 p.m.
Wed	Eat only from 12 p.m.–8 p.m.	Eat normally	Eat normally	24-hour fast
Thu	Eat only from 12 p.m.–8 p.m.	24-hour fast	24-hour fast	Eat only from 12 p.m.–8 p.m.
Fri	Eat only from 12 p.m.–8 p.m.	Eat normally	Eat normally	Eat only from 12 p.m.–8 p.m.
Sat	Eat only from 12 p.m.–8 p.m.	Eat normally	24-hour fast	Eat only from 12 p.m.–8 p.m.
Sun	Eat only from 12 p.m.–8 p.m.	Eat normally	Eat normally	Eat only from 12 p.m.–8 p.m.

Summary of Common Fasting Patterns

The flexibility of intermittent fasting is one of the things that makes it sustainable for the long term. You can fast no matter what type of diet you follow, and you can choose whatever fasting pattern works for you. I consider it a gift to eaters everywhere!

That said, lots of options can be overwhelming, especially if you're used to traditional diets with strict rules and limitations. There's value in having restrictions, especially when you're starting out. So if you want a short list to pick from, here are your top three choices.

Option 1: A 16:8 time-restricted eating window

Eat within an eight hour window every day. It's probably best to note the time you finish dinner, and count back eight hours from there—that's your starting time. Don't consume any calories the rest of the time. Water, black coffee, and unsweetened tea are okay to have. Keep this pattern on the weekend, too, if you can. Plan morning activities to keep you busy, especially if your family is home eating breakfast. Stick with this fast for six weeks. If you miss a day here and there, keep going. If, after a couple of weeks, the pattern feels easy, or you're just not hungry for your first meal, lengthen your fast by two hours and see how that goes. On the flip side, if at the end of six weeks this daily pattern is not working for you, consider options 2 or 3.

Option 2: A 24-hour fast

Pick a day that you want to fast. On that day, you will eat dinner only. The night before, make sure to eat a normal dinner at a reasonable hour, and don't snack afterward. Don't stuff yourself at dinner, because it may make your fast harder the next day. Stick to high-fat foods and quality protein for that meal, and avoid anything sugary or starchy. Before you go to sleep, put a sticky note on your bathroom mirror to remind you when you wake up in the morning that you are fasting that day. If you forget, you're liable to eat breakfast and miss your fasting opportunity! Enjoy your fast for the day, have dinner in the evening, and eat normally the rest of the week. Seven days later, do the 24-hour fast again. Practice this for six weeks. If you love it and want to do more, great—choose a second fasting day during the week. Eventually, if you want, you can choose a third. If, on the other hand, you don't like this pattern at all after six weeks, consider options 1 or 3.

Option 3: The 5:2 fast

Pick two days on which to eat only 25 percent of the amount you normally eat. So if you normally aim for 2000 calories, that'll be 500 calories for your fasting days. That's a very small vegetable salad with some cheese or a little protein, and oil-based dressing. Or, that's half a piece of salmon with a side of green vegetables and half an avocado. Aside from that meal, don't eat anything else that day. Eat normally the rest of the week until your second fasting day, and then eat only 25 percent again on that day. For simplicity's sake, it's good to keep the same two days every week, but if you have a social invitation one week that falls on your fasting day, just move your fast to another day. Stick with this for six weeks. You may find that it's easier to go without eating on your fasting days than to eat the small meal (many people do). If so, skip the meal! If after six weeks you really don't like this pattern, try options 1 or 2.

Time-Restricted Eating

If you are new to intermittent fasting, I recommend you start with time-restricted eating. In this pattern, you eat all your food within a specific window of time each day. Most people start out skipping breakfast and eating dinner at a reasonable hour, i.e., a couple of hours before bedtime (no snacking afterward). If you eat lunch at 12 p.m. and dinner before 8 p.m., you've got yourself a 16-hour fast! This is commonly called the "16:8," because you fast for 16 hours (ideally sleeping half the time), and eat for 8 hours. You're permitted snacks during your eating window, though many people find they're not hungry enough to eat more than two meals in 8 hours' time. Your appetite will likely diminish over time, so be attentive to your needs and don't try to cram in meals when you're not hungry.

The "skip breakfast" schedule is a common one, but it's not the only way to practice this fast. If you are someone for whom breakfast is essential, you can still do the 16:8—just shift your eating window to start earlier in the day. For you, a 9 a.m.-5 p.m. eating window may work best. Alternatively, if your business or social life means that dinners usually happen late, then start your fast later in the day so you have time in the evening to accommodate your last meal. You may find that a 2 p.m.-10 p.m. eating window is the right fit for you. Your goal is simply to have 16 hours of fasting time. You muscles will be relying on fats for energy and sparing glucose for the brain. Insulin levels will have been low for 10 hours or more, making fat more available as an energy source and allowing ketone production to proceed.

With 16 hours of fasting, you'll have achieved a lot of the metabolic changes—ketosis, insulin reduction, growth hormone spike—that you are seeking. It is two-thirds of a day, and it's a great amount of time to be in the fasted state. That said, if you're challenged to meet the 16-hour fasting goal, then simply start with less and work your way up. Soon, you will find that the biggest obstacle to fasting is a psychological one. Start with a 12-hour fast if that's what you feel you can do right now (and remember, eight hours are sleep time), and simply delay your first meal by an hour every few days. I believe you'll be able to work up to a 16-hour fast in no time.

One of the benefits of time-restricted eating is that it may work in synergy with your circadian rhythm. This is the "internal clock" that responds to light and dark and influences physiological signals such as sleepiness, wakefulness, and hunger. There's good evidence that eating during daylight hours is best for our metabolic health, whereas eating at night (when our internal clock wants us to be sleeping) is not so good. If you think about it, for most of human history, eating had to be done during the day because there was no artificial light by which to eat at nighttime. This pattern works with the natural circadian rhythm.

Another benefit of time-restricted eating is that it eliminates the common problem of late-night snacking. When your eating window closes at 8 p.m., there's no peeking in the cabinets for a nibble just before bed. The rules are clear: no eating outside your eating window, which means dinner is the last eating moment of the day. At night, herbal teas are a very good treat.

Interview with Ashley Colpaart, age 36

Type of fast: Time-restricted eating

Ashley is the CEO of a food technology company that connects food entrepreneurs with commercial kitchen space. She is also a registered dietitian and has a PhD in food science and food safety from Colorado State University.

Q: *Why did you start fasting?*

A: I stumbled upon it. My sister who lives in California posted about it at a time when I was struggling with my weight. I knew it was a matter of stress as I was trying to finish my dissertation and start a company, and I wasn't managing my weight well. I was searching for things to turn my weight gain around—like, I did a month of yoga—and I was open to trying new things because I was just stuck. That night I downloaded the app Zero, which helps you keep track of your fasts. It has a science section with hours of videos by fasting researchers—Panda, Longo, Ruth Patterson—and I become really intrigued. Especially as a registered dietitian with a background in science, it grabbed me. Then I joined the Facebook group *Delay, Don't Deny*. This community...was extra supportive, and people who had struggled with their weight and other ailments for years were seeing results..,and quickly! As a dietitian and a public health professional you always tell people there is no "magic bullet" for weight loss, and yet here these people were having this dramatic change in their bodies and their overall health. They were empowered and able to take control of something that seemed futile.

As for me, [while fasting,] I lost 15 pounds in two months! And I started gaining lean body mass. My clothes started fitting better and I threw out my worn-out stretchy jeans. I don't even fit into the original wedding dress I bought for my wedding a year later. And I haven't changed anything else—I still eat exactly the same, I just do time-restricted eating. It's super easy, empowering, and fits with my lifestyle. It is a "way of eating," not a diet.

Q: *What's does your fasting pattern look like?*

A: I aim for 16 to 20 fasting hours per day. I close my eating window by 8 p.m. every night. Sixteen hours of fasting is my minimum every day, and sometimes I'll do 18, and if I'm feeling really good I'll do 20. So, I aim for 16 to 20 fasting hours per day.

I skip breakfast every day and I only drink black coffee and water during my fasting window. I don't do anything that would spur insulin release: I don't put cream in my coffee, I don't chew gum, etc. Decreasing insulin gets me into mild ketosis every day, meaning my body is switching to burning fat for fuel. I get into ketosis pretty easily now, having been intermittent fasting for four months.

Q: *What do you eat when you're not fasting?*

A: I open my eating window with a snack, like almonds, hard boiled eggs, or yogurt. Dinner may be vegetable and tofu curry with rice, and a Noosa yogurt for dessert. I also drink red wine in my window. If I feel like eating something when my window is open I do. I don't deny myself the foods I want to eat.

Q: *Has it impacted your relationships?*

A: My husband does it with me: we just don't eat breakfast anymore, and often don't eat lunch either during the week, and we go out to eat in the evenings. We eat the things we want. On the weekends, we don't eat until 2 p.m. We also go to the gym in a fasted state. For work, I try to avoid scheduling breakfast or lunch meetings. It is pretty easy to build your schedule and social life around this lifestyle and if I feel like I am missing out, I will just open my window earlier and do a longer fast the next day. It's flexible.

Q: *Is there anything about intermittent fasting that really surprised you, either in your own practice or in your research?*

A: When you first tell people you're doing it they think you're crazy. They often say they can't go 3 to 4 hours without eating or they feel terrible. I felt that way the first few days, but what was astonishing to me is how quickly you get through that—and you begin to feel lighter, better, stronger. My energy levels improved. My mental clarity improved. I used to crash in the middle of the day, and that doesn't happen now.

I was also surprised by the community—how much of a lifestyle this is, versus a diet. Usually we're too restrictive [with weight loss diets], and we make people feel like they're failing when they can't stick to the diet. This, on the other hand, is empowering. You say to yourself "I can eat cake tonight at the birthday party, I'm just not opening my eating window until 5 p.m." So I guess I am surprised at how liberating it is, and at the same time how in control you feel.

The most intriguing part to me is the emerging science on the autophagy side of things, as well as hormone control. Insulin regulates blood glucose and storage and metabolism of energy. Controlling your hormones is a super powerful thing because it is regulating everything. Bringing down insulin levels is very important, but most people don't ever bring down insulin because they are always eating. Really the only time they're not is when they're sleeping.

Growth hormone release starts at 16 hours of fasting and spikes between 18 and 20 hours. The neat part of fasting is in gaining lean muscle mass. People think if you're not eating you're going to lose muscle, but actually, the opposite happens. My whole physique and body type has changed. People in the *Delay, Don't Deny* group have seen their stretch marks and wrinkles go away. It's from the cell turnover that happens when you're in the fasted state thanks to autophagy. People post their before and after pictures and it's really unbelievable.

Q: *Why do you think dietitians and nutrition professionals discourage fasting, or simply don't consider it as a legitimate strategy for patients seeking weight loss?*

A: I think we are anchored or bound by confirmation bias of what we believe, that "calories in/calories out" is the way, because we've been trained to believe this. There's a cultural influence of three meals a day, and this notion that breakfast is the most important, and if you don't eat often your metabolism will slow down. Shifting that set of beliefs... will take time. I think more studies and clinical trials will help. When more people get weight loss results and get their life back from intermittent fasting...then that will get reactions from providers who want their clients to succeed. But, there's not a lot of money to be made from fasting in the food industry... and I would guess that will be part of the criticism of if fasting gets more popular.

Q: *What would you recommend to people who are considering intermittent fasting?*

A: It's just so simple. Start by reading one of the many books on intermittent fasting. I suggest Dr. Jason Fung's *Obesity Code* and *Delay, Don't Deny* by Gin Stephens.... I think it's going to be the way that people get a hold of their life. It's a new lease on life. And I think it's simple enough that it's sustainable.

If you are severely overweight and you move to a 16:8 daily fasting pattern, I think you can drop a lot of weight. As you start getting thinner you have to shorten that window to keep losing weight, and if you're trying to get real results and not just maintenance, you also have to cut out refined sugars and alcohol and eat healthy, nutrient-dense foods during your eating window.

Q: *Do you think you'll continue with intermittent fasting forever?*

A: Well I guess "forever" is a hard word to say, but it'll probably be something I incorporate into my lifestyle for the long haul, maybe taking breaks for vacation. I'm getting a lot of value outside of just the weight loss, because I feel so much better!

Lengthening a Daily Fast

Whether you start with a fast of 16 hours or work your way up to it, you may find after a couple of weeks that you can go longer. If you fast in the early part of the day, you'll notice that you're not always hungry when your first mealtime comes around. You may be excited about your progress and feeling empowered, which may give you the motivation to wait another two hours before breaking your fast. After having skipped breakfast every day without trouble, you'll want to challenge yourself to skip lunch some days too—especially if you were someone who thought you could never manage to skip breakfast even once! Without even realizing, you might make it to dinnertime and discover you haven't eaten since yesterday. This is how people come to dive deeper into the daily fasting pattern, shortening their daily eating window to six, four, or even two hours. The 18:6 or 20:4 are quite popular and relatively easy to maintain, at least during the weekdays. Fat burning is quite high in the 18 to 24 hour period of your fast, so it is worth shooting for that length of time on many or most fasting days. If you don't have a lot of lean body mass (e.g., if you're female and/or you have a high body fat ratio) then you may find more fat-burning success extending your fast to 36 hours.

Some people follow the One Meal A Day (OMAD) pattern, which is akin to a 22- or 23-hour fast every single day (23:1), depending on how long you give yourself to eat your one meal. If you're going out to dinner and having appetizers and an entree, for instance, then you may not want to squeeze the whole experience into one hour, so you'll give yourself two hours. Conversely, some people are super strict about their fasting times and stick to a timed eating window every day, at the same time, with no exceptions. If that's your style, then go for it, but don't feel you need to be so strict. It's not going to mess up your ketosis or impede your fat loss if you fast less one day or eat at a different time another day. As mentioned previously, the exact number of hours to achieve a given level of ketosis will vary from person to person and will be influenced by your previous meals, level of exercise or energy spent that day, and other factors.

One of the major benefits of eating once a day is that it is simple and doesn't require you to think about an eating schedule. You get back a lot of time and mental energy that would have otherwise been spent on figuring out what and when to eat.

The downside to OMAD is that it lacks variability in energy intake, which can lead to weight plateau. Think about it: if you eat only once a day, you'll probably be eating about the same number of calories day in and day out, and you'll be eating fewer calories than you would if you ate multiple meals per day. This looks a lot like a calorie-restricted diet—the very kind that cause weight plateau. For this reason, one meal a day is a good pattern to stick with for weight maintenance. If you are eating one meal a day and hit a plateau when you still want to be losing weight, go ahead and switch things up. You can add a 36- or 48-hour fast into your week, or a three day fast every other week, for example, and include a couple of days where you eat more than one meal so you can have a much more varied energy intake.

What's important is that you get a command of intermittent fasting and include it in your life in ways that suit you. The precise timing of meals or fasting windows that will lead to "optimal" fat loss matters less than just getting some fasting time in, period. I recommend finding a pattern that fits with your schedule so meals are convenient, and fasting time doesn't disrupt your life. Choose something you will be able to maintain consistently. When needed, make adjustments or vary the schedule to continue to achieve your goals.

Jonathan Deutsch, age 41

Type of fast: One meal a day

Jonathan is a professor in the Center for Food and Hospitality Management and Department of Nutrition Sciences at Drexel University. He runs the Drexel Food Lab, focused on good food product development.

Q: *Why did you start intermittent fasting?*

A: I participated in a weight loss study with the National Institutes of Health (NIH) that started in April 2015. It was a three-year study focused on weight maintenance. We had weekly weigh-ins, some nutrition education, calorie tracking, and exercise tracking. My starting weight was 333 pounds and my calorie budget was 1800 cal/day. They gave suggestions and sample meal plans with foods like oatmeal for breakfast, turkey sandwiches for lunch, and broiled fish for dinner. I started getting very frustrated because I'm a chef and I like to eat everything! I knew the foods I wanted would blow my calorie budget. Also, I am naturally not hungry in the morning, but I had it in my head that breakfast is the most important meal of the day so I was forcing myself to eat in the morning, and sometimes by the afternoon I would blow my whole calorie budget, and then be hungry the rest of the day.

I also love to have big dinners out. Often I would only have, say, 400 calories left by dinner, and I just felt frustrated because I couldn't eat the foods I wanted. It felt like every meal was pretty disappointing. I love eating! Eating is one of my main motivations to live. Honestly, if I had to give that up, I just felt like I would rather deal with the health consequences.

So I just decided to experiment; I thought, "What if I don't eat all day and then just eat a nice dinner?"—1800 calories is a nice dinner! I could get three or four courses, and even if I wanted a burger or steak sandwich I could still eat that—it would fit into the 1800 calories if I skipped eating the rest of the day, and then I wouldn't have to eat diet food. I didn't know anything about intermittent fasting—I came to this on my own.

Q: *What does your fasting pattern look like?*

A: I drink coffee all day, I do put milk and sugar in it sometimes but not always. If I get really famished I'll have an apple or orange midday. I'm not crazy about it. I'm totally fine if my colleagues are all going to lunch, I have no problem saying, "I don't eat lunch anymore." That's fine. I try to do one meal a day, and I like dinner because there's less time left and once I start eating I can just keep going. I'm sure I could eat 5000 to 6000 calories in a day, easily. By the time I eat dinner there are only a few hours left, so it limits my eating, whereas if I eat Sunday brunch I'm just going to eat all day.

I'm not as austere about it on the weekends. It's hard because I'm home and I'm the main cook. If I make pancakes on the weekend, I will probably have half of one. If we're traveling and at a hotel, I might just take a walk, or stay in the room while my family goes to the breakfast buffet.

Q: *How long have you been intermittent fasting?*

A: Three years now. I've lost a lot of weight. I got to 249 pounds, so I lost 85 pounds from my original weight. Then I went back up to 275. They say it's good to be up 10 percent from your lowest weight because if you're hovering around your lowest then you are likely to rebound. I'm 20 percent up from my lowest now. That was a good realization too, to stick with it for maintenance. A lot of diet books say, "Do this plan, lose the weight, and then you can add things back." I know that won't work for me. I know I have to do this forever. I think about it through a disabilities framework—other people can eat three meals a day and not get fat. I can't do that. That frame is a lot more helpful to me.

Q: *Any suggestions for people who want to try intermittent fasting?*

A: I have finally found something that works for me. I know a lot of people who have good intentions [and suggest other approaches for weight loss], like snacking on nuts. But I can't succeed like that. That said, if you can't imagine ever doing this because you know you would be lightheaded, hangry, etc., then don't do it. I know for instance that my wife could not do it. She feels unwell when she fasts. So if this isn't the right thing for you, don't do it. But it is the thing that really works for me.

Fast a Couple Times Each Week

You don't have to stick to a time-restricted eating window every day in order to practice intermittent fasting. If your work responsibilities mean you'll have to join colleagues for dinner at varying times, or if you have an active social life that includes dining out, then it may be tough for you to keep a daily eating window. Don't worry—you can organize fasts on days of the week when your schedule permits. Part of the beauty of intermittent fasting is its flexibility.

On the popular 5:2 diet, you eat normally five days a week and fast for two days each week. If not eating for an entire day sounds intimidating, keep in mind that you don't have to exclude all meals on a given day. You just have to arrange for a fasting period of a full 24 hours. For example, if one of your fasting days is Thursday, you can eat dinner on Wednesday night, wrapping up by 8 p.m. You fast Thursday morning and afternoon, and plan for dinner to start at around 8 p.m. Thursday night. That way, you'll fast from dinner Wednesday until dinner Thursday, for a total of 24 hours. Do the same for your other fasting day, from dinner to dinner. You'll have fasted 48 hours that week! Eat normally the rest of the week, and repeat the pattern every week.

Pick fasting days that makes sense for your life. You might pick two days that are always hectic at work, because you like being busy while you're fasting. Plan to do some errands or exercise in the evening, and come home properly hungry for your meal those nights. Or maybe you have a day each week that calls out to you as the day you like to rest. This could even be associated with a social or religious practice, such as keeping Sabbath on Saturday, or resting from work on Sunday. You may discover that a fast, or "rest" from eating, is a nice addition to your practice on that day. The important thing is not which days you choose; it's that you choose them, and stick with them week after week.

If you really want to hit the ground running, try a 24-hour fast three days per week. Fast on Monday, Wednesday, and Friday (or whatever schedule works for you). As you get accustomed to the pattern—and your shrinking waist size—you'll find it surprisingly doable. Another riff on this pattern is called alternate-day fasting, and it is as simple as it sounds: eat one day, fast the next. There is a nice rhythm to it. A lot of the benefits we attribute to intermittent fasting come from studies using alternate-day fasting in both animals and humans. It's a good approach from a metabolic standpoint, but it is somewhat impractical because there are an odd number of days every week—which means your fasting days will change every week. It's a lot easier, I think, to pick three fasting days a week and stick with them.

Some versions of full-day fasts allow for a small meal that pro-vides about 25 percent of your normal calorie needs (i.e., about 400 to 600 calories). This is not going to undo all the benefits of the fast, but it can be tricky to consume food on your fasting days. First, it's hard to gauge the number of calories in a meal, and it's very easy to eat more than you think you're eating. It can also be a slippery slope—once you start eating, you may just want to continue, and before you know it, your fasting day has turned into an eating day. But, it is nice to have a backup plan in case the fast is feeling particularly difficult that day. So, take the option to have the small amount of food if you think it will help you get more fasting time overall.

Beth Zupec-Kania, age 59

Type of fast: Time-restricted eating and 36-hour
weekly fast, plus a ketogenic diet

Any book that includes a discussion of ketosis should devote some space to the work of Beth Zupec-Kania, registered dietitian nutritionist and ketogenic specialist for the Charlie Foundation for Ketogenic Therapies. Beth's focus is on treating epilepsy and other neurological disorders, certain cancers, and genetic-metabolic disorders with ketogenic diet therapy. She has worked with hundreds of people all over the world on the ketogenic diet, and follows one herself. I interviewed Beth about her personal experience with intermittent fasting and following a ketogenic diet. Learn more about her at www.bethzupeckania.com.

Q: *Why do you practice intermittent fasting?*

A: I practice intermittent fasting because I have experienced the great benefits that are reported. I started doing it in solidarity with my clients prior to starting ketogenic diet therapy. I felt like I it would be easier for them if we could do it together, and it's become a weekly practice for me.

So much of the difficulty of fasting is the emotional aspect of it, the fear of "starving yourself," but also the loss of the social event of eating with someone. So it's easier to fast with a buddy to replace that social aspect. Once you get into a routine of regular fasting, you realize what a powerful therapy it is. My schedule of fasting starts after dinner on Sunday and continues through Monday. I go to yoga on Tuesday morning and then have lunch afterward to end the fast (36 hours). I felt great once I let go of the feeling of depriving myself of food and the social aspect of eating, and instead focused on the physical and mental benefits that I gained with fasting.

As an almost 60-year-old woman, intermittent fasting and maintaining a ketogenic diet have helped me maintain the same weight as when I was 25! I don't weigh myself; actually, my scale is in the basement. I can just tell from the way my clothes fit. This style of eating helps avoid the typical weight gain that many adults experience as they age.

Q: *What does your diet look like when you're in your eating phase?*

A: I eat a gluten-free, mostly plant-based diet. I only eat two meals a day, and one of those meals is always vegan. Lunch, for example, is a sprouted (seed) salad with sunflower/pumpkin seeds and avocado oil dressing (homemade). Another favorite meal of mine is a blended smoothie with olive and medium-chain triglyceride (MCT) oils, sprouted protein powder, water, and unsweetened cocoa, with green banana or berries as the carbohydrate.

I spend more time on my evening meal when I have time to cook and my husband is here with me; that's our daily time together. The second meal is usually fish, and occasionally animal protein, and I do eat dairy, mostly butter, ghee, and small amounts of aged cheese and heavy cream.

My first meal of the day is at 1 p.m., but sometimes I fast a bit longer. I tell myself 1 p.m. is my eating time, but in actuality I wait until I have the sensation of stomach growling, which is a good way to know that you are truly hungry. Dinner is sometime between 6 and 7 p.m. I cut myself off at 8 p.m., so no snacks at all after that.

In addition to the intermittent daily fasting, I do the 24 to 36 hour fast once a week; usually from dinner on Sunday to lunch on Tuesday, but if I have company, I will move it over to another day.

Q: *You seem very committed to intermittent fasting. How do you stick with it?*

A: It's happened over time. I have been doing intermittent fasting for four years, and following a ketogenic diet for eight years. I've learned a lot from my clients during that time. We can talk together about the "aha" moment, the "I get this" feeling. It feels so good, it truly is good for us [adults], and I really believe it slows the aging process!

Q: *Do you recommend fasting to help people get in ketosis for weight loss?*

A: It's standard practice for people starting ketogenic therapy—adults usually start with a fast. Ketosis depresses appetite, which gives them appetite control. Some of my clients have told me that it's the first time in their life that they aren't constantly thinking about food. Fasting can boost that effect, especially for people who have days where they overeat or are inactive. Many adults find a ketogenic lifestyle to be the only method for maintaining weight loss long-term.

Q: *Do you ever eat sweets?*

A: I honestly don't eat sweets at all. It's funny because my husband is a sweets eater. I recently bought him a cheesecake because it's his favorite dessert, but I didn't have any of it. I do enjoy dark chocolate (92 percent) and sometimes have a piece as a "dessert."

Q: *What's the toughest part of following the ketogenic diet?*

A: Wine was my hardest food to cut back on! But I found Dry Farm Wines, which has less than 1 gram of carb per bottle of wine. Instead of drinking two or three glasses of wine, I drink one glass at most. And I love vegetables, and always have a large raw vegetable salad for dinner or with dinner with 4 to 5 tablespoons of olive oil dressing.

Q: *What would you say are the differences between ketogenic dieting and fasting?*

A: Intermittent fasting of 12 or 16 hours a day is easiest for most people to adapt to initially and quickly. And once you adapt physically and emotionally to intermittent fasting, longer fasting periods are achievable. Meanwhile, adopting a well-balanced ketogenic diet will take more time and research. "Keto flu" is common when adjusting to a keto diet; generally, my clients who gradually adopt a keto diet over several weeks don't complain of this.

Q: *What piece of advice would you give to someone who's just started out with an intermittent fasting practice?*

A: Find a buddy to do this with you. It will make this much easier to manage, even if you just text each other. Pick a day and time to start together and check in with each other every few hours.

Interview with Douglas Park, age 33

Type of fast: One meal a day and alternate-day fasting

Douglas Park is the owner of the craft spirits label Tokki Soju, and is an avid intermittent fasting practitioner.

Q: *What does your intermittent fasting practice look like?*

A: I alternate between two patterns. Ten years ago, I started eating only one meal a day. Then six months ago, I also started fasting completely every other day.

Q: *Why did you start fasting?*

A: At the time, I was obsessed with going to the gym. I was reading something written by a famous bodybuilder whose name I can't remember. His theory was that our body has not evolved since caveman days, and he recommended not eating three meals a day. I tried it, and I realized right off the bat that my mind was clearer and I could function better, and then I never went back to eating regularly.

When I hit 31, I really started to experience slowing of my metabolism. I was gaining weight pretty easily. So I starting running three or four miles, five times a week, but I did not see any progress. And I hate running! So I thought, I'm going to just cut back on eating. That's when I started doing the alternate-day fasting, and with that, I saw significant results immediately.

Q: *Do you get hungry?*

A: Whenever I feel hungry, I drink two cups of water, and most of the time after the water I don't feel hungry anymore. I would say that six or eight hours after eating is probably when I feel the most hungry. Usually I eat at night, so I usually feel hungry when I wake up. Then it goes away after water and coffee.

Q: *Do you consume anything during your fast?*

A: Just water and black coffee and tea.

Q: *Why do you keep it up?*

A: Eating every other day has been very liberating for me, compared to doing next-to-no carbs [for weight maintenance] because my favorite foods are pizza and pasta. Also, when you go out, it's very hard to be in a group setting to order and not have carbs. Now that I eat every other day, I just eat what I want. Then I fast for 36 to 48 hours at a time.

Q: *What would you say are the biggest challenges, and which things are easier than you thought they'd be?*

A: Eating every other day is very manageable. I don't feel like I have to put much effort into it. It would be harder if I didn't have the flexibility to schedule my work time, but it's not a struggle for me because I own my own business and set my own schedule.

Q: *Do you have any tips for people new to the practice?*

A: I would say get friendly with tea. That helps tremendously. Drinking water by itself is so boring! Also, I personally can't drink coffee past 3 p.m. because it affects my sleep. So when I'm not eating, I'll often drink tea and it's a great way to get through your day without feeling bored. I also highly recommend eating lots of fat. It just makes you full better than any other stuff. I don't shy away from butter, pork belly, and stuff like that.

Infrequent Fasts

Fasting on a regular schedule helps you establish a routine and makes fasting a part of your life. Sometimes it's nice to go deeper into the practice every so often. Maybe you want to schedule a three-day or even a five-day fast once a month or every other month to amplify the benefits. Not everyone is going to be able (or excited) to do this, and that's perfectly okay! Even if you don't schedule something of the sort, keep your mind open to possibilities. For example, if you have a week of heavy eating with friends in town or a family gathering, you might be ready to try a few days of fasting the next week. If you do a multi-day fast, you can always consider the option of simply having 25 percent of your normal calories on fasting days.

As I've said before, you really can choose what works for you. If you are like most Westerners, you have spent the majority of your life eating three meals a day, every day, and more when the opportunity presents itself. Any additional time spent fasting is a gift to your body, mind, and soul. If you stick to time-restricted eating for your regular fasting practice and pick just one full day a month for a dedicated fast on top of that, that's a very nice bonus. It all adds up.

Yearly fasts are another option. If you are fasting to lose weight, then a once a year fast is probably not going to help you achieve your long-term goals. That said, a yearly fasting practice can be very beneficial as a meditation or time of reflection, distinct from the practice you maintain of fasting for weight loss. Many religious and cultural traditions designate particular times of the year for fasting with the goal of slowing down and resting, reflecting, and rejuvenating. In our modern, hectic times, a yearly fast can be a very powerful relaxation tool. Like a vacation, a yearly fasting practice of even a few days can offer a significant sense of peace and rejuvenation.

Not surprisingly, a common practice on wellness retreats is for participants to fast or eat very lightly. This may be combined with a spiritual or mindfulness practice such as meditation, or a physical one such as yoga. Going on a retreat where fasting is a part of the program is a smart way to familiarize yourself with a meditative fasting practice. These programs provide a structured day and ongoing guidance from retreat leaders so that practitioners are not left on their own. There's a community of people sharing the experience together, many of whom are new to the practice themselves. This sort of environment makes it easy to go along with the new eating patterns and other practices, even if those things would be unfamiliar in your home setting.

Long-Term Fasts

There are extreme cases of medically supervised fasts for obese patients lasting many months. The longest recorded fast was undertaken by an obese man who fasted for over a year and lost 276 pounds! Of course, this unique case is often referred to as a way to illustrate the point that humans can survive on their body fat, and not put forth as a treatment option for the average person. Fasting for such a length of time can be incredibly dangerous, and the man who completed this fast was under constant supervision and provided with medical support when needed. What's important to remember about fasting is that it is cumulative: fast for two days every week, and keep it up for a year—by the end of the year you'll have fasted for 104 days!

Another way to look at the world record for "longest fast" is to consider the world record for just about anything. According to the Guinness Book of World Records, the longest swim in open water was 139.8 miles in the Adriatic Sea. It's absolutely impossible for the average person to swim that far in open sea and survive! But it is food for thought: if that guy can swim 140 miles, maybe you and I and the average Joe can train enough to swim one mile at sea, and practice swimming reasonable distances as a healthy exercise. And if that other guy can fast for an entire year, maybe you and I and the average Joe can fast for a day or two every week and reap the same benefits over time.

My Ramadan Experience

My first experience with fasting was during the once-a-year observance of the Muslim holiday of Ramadan in 2011. Ramadan spans 30 days and moves through the lunar calendar so that it falls at a different time every year. Observers consume no food or water during the daylight hours of Ramadan, having nourishment only when the sun is down. If you're in a place where the days are long in the summer and short in the winter, then the number of hours you fast will change as Ramadan moves through the seasons. In 2011, Ramadan fell in August. I was in NYC, which meant the fast would be from about 3:30 a.m. to 8:30 p.m., or 17 hours a day. This is about as long as it gets. (To be sure, Ramadan is an important holiday in the Muslim world and there is much more to it than abstaining from food and drink. I cannot say I observed Ramadan itself—only that I chose to follow the pattern of a Ramadan fast during that same time.)

I was fortunate to have Muslim friends who were familiar with Ramadan support me through the experience. Without them, I probably would not have been able to complete the fast. The days in August were long and very hot. After three days of fasting I realized lack of food was not my biggest challenge—I was rarely hungry and I mostly forgot about food. But I was extremely thirsty. Now I don't recommend fasting without water (in fact, I recommend a lot of water during your fast), but I was following in the spirit of Ramadan which does not allow water during fasting time. For this being my first fasting experience, the lack of water sure put things in perspective.

Fasting for Ramadan put a lot of things in perspective for me. My days got quieter. My mind slowed, and I was able to consider things I'd wanted to think deeply about but never did before because I couldn't stop my attention from jumping around. I noticed other things I'd never noticed before, like the fact that some friends didn't want to spend time with me if we couldn't consume food or drink. Some did, and we met for walks in the park, a visit to a museum, or quiet conversation at home. Some didn't mind if I joined them for a meal and didn't eat myself. But this experience made me realize that the act of consumption is often a gateway to socializing. So many social events revolve around going out to eat or drink, especially in a city environment—there's dinner, brunch, a cocktail after work. Because of this, if you choose not to consume, you're often left alone and feeling lonely. I asked my Muslim friends how they handled these situations, given they had much more experience with it. Their advice was sound: try to have a good-natured attitude about it, don't ask friends who aren't comfortable with it to accommodate your new habits during your fasting period, and realize that it's only for a short time. "You can join your friends for meals without concern the rest of the year," they said. "Brunch will still be there when you're done with Ramadan."

After that, my approach to food changed. I was calmer and more comfortable when I got hungry, and patient enough to wait for mealtimes instead of reaching for the nearest snack to quell the sensation. And I had always believed that would be impossible.

Breaking a Fast

People always want to know what they can "eat" on their fast. That's easy: Nothing. Eat nothing! You are fasting. That's the point.

You cannot drink anything with calories (juice, soda, "vitamin water," coconut water, etc.), nor can you drink "diet beverages" without calories (diet soda, diet vitamin water, diet anything). You cannot have gum, sucking candy, breath mints, Tic Tacs, or anything of the sort. If you're following the sort of plan that allows for a small meal (approximately 500 calories) once a day, then you will eat only that meal, and won't have food outside of that.

You must, however, drink a good amount of water (see Chapter 8). You can have also have unflavored carbonated water. And you can have coffee and tea, unsweetened (including fake sweeteners), and without milk.

How to Take Care of Yourself with Intermittent Fasting

Fasting for short periods of time is safe and simple for healthy adults. No special preparation or changes to your daily activities are required. You just choose periods of time not to eat, and go about your normal business while fasting. Once you start doing research you'll find dozens of websites and videos detailing "secret tips for optimizing your fast," from drinking apple cider vinegar to supplementing with branched chain amino acids (BCAAs) or medium-chain triglyceride (MCT) oil. But there's no need to make this more complicated than it needs to be! While none of these tips are harmful, they're also not necessary—and they can create a lot of extra work and confusion, making fasting seem much more difficult than it really is. The more complicated it is, the less likely you are to stick with it. It's best to keep things simple.

In your research, you might also come across articles obsessing over electrolyte imbalance and scary information about something called "refeeding syndrome." If I were new to fasting and had no background in metabolic science, I would be turned off to the whole thing. But these are not important concerns for healthy adults who practice intermittent fasting and eat an adequate diet otherwise. There are some good practices for taking care of yourself on your fast, which we'll review in this chapter. For example, drinking broth is a good practice for multi-day fasts. You can take some supplements if you notice they make you feel better. But it's really not essential to do any of that. People all over the world fast all the time without consuming special foods or supplements to prepare, and do just fine.

Interview with Megan Ramos

Subject: Therapeutic fasting

Q: *Tell us who you are and what you do.*

A: I'm a clinical researcher, and cofounder and CEO of the Intensive Dietary Management program along with Dr. Jason Fung. IDM is a therapeutic fasting program. I run the business, and train providers on how to use intermittent fasting with their patients. I also write books and speak on podcasts on the subject of fasting.

When I was younger, I was what you'd call "skinny fat" [skinny, but with metabolic health problems common to people who are overweight]. I had fatty liver disease and PCOS. For some reason, doctors didn't care about body composition; they just cared about the number on the scale. I was able to stay "skinny fat" because I did time-restricted eating without even meaning to. I was in school studying, and I just usually forgot to eat. When I was done with school, it was important to start functioning "like an adult," which meant eating three proper meals and three snacks a day, and never going to bed hungry. So then, I became "fat fat" and diabetic!

Jason Fung started becoming interested in fasting because of some conversations with friends who practiced fasting for religious reasons. So he talked with me about it, and we tried it on me.

Q: *What do you love most about your job?*

A: Making people better! That's the best part because I had totally lost faith. You think doctors are supposed to help people, but doctors are taught to manage disease, not improve it. When I was doing research, I was monitoring people with kidney disease, and all I did was watch people die. Whenever they came in for their appointments, they just got more medication, and were told they were a little worse. But never, ever did someone get better.

Now I come in to work and every day someone is off their meds. Every day, someone loses weight. Every day everyone loses weight! Everyone gets better. We're giving people their lives back. And this whole group—the type 2 diabetics—has been written off by the medical community. But it doesn't have to be that way. We can make them better.

Q: *What are some of the most common results you see in patients who keep a fasting practice?*

A: Body composition change. I won't say "weight loss." It's body fat reduction and lean mass growth. Our patients lose body fat, but they gain lean mass and muscle mass. A lot of women who have osteoporosis improve it or get rid of it altogether. We see total reversal of diabetes. We have patients come to us on insulin with consistently high blood sugar, and we see their blood sugars normalize, and they can stop taking medication. We see a dramatic improvement in fatty liver disease or a reversal of it. More than half the time, their blood pressure improves and they're able to come off those meds as well. People report extreme mental clarity—brain fog is totally lifted. We see increased performance, whether mental or physical or both—which is so amazing, because you get increased productivity.

Q: *What sort of a fasting course do people follow in your program?*

A: The program varies for everyone. Some people come in on 100 units of insulin and we give them a super aggressive fasting regimen. Some people's blood sugars just won't budge. I have one patient who is on his fifty-sixth day of a water fast because his sugars just won't budge. And then there are people exactly like him who do a 24-hour fast and they just stop eating potatoes and their sugars become perfect and they never need insulin again. We really nail in that this is a therapeutic treatment, and you have to commit. An analogy would be chemotherapy—it's a serious treatment, and you don't do it halfway. With therapeutic fasting, you commit to it and you do it. It depends how compliant they want to be. We find that within six months, most people are off of their diabetic meds.

Q: *I know a lot of your patients do extended fasts of a week or more. What sort of supervision do you recommend for a fast of that length?*

A: We see them a lot. We do blood work once or twice a week, and I may see them two times spread out in the week, like on a Monday and Thursday. Most people commonly do up to 14 days of fasting and we see them one to two times per week, and they get weekly blood work done.

Q: *I've heard you say the benefits of fasting accumulate the more you do it. In your view, is there real value to doing shorter fasts (e.g., time-restricted eating, or a 24-hour fast two or three times a week) as well?*

A: Absolutely. The bottom line is we all need to do time-restricted eating. I think if people just didn't snack late at night, a large portion of these metabolic problems would disappear. Even if someone can never get off their meds, even if their sugars are still terrible—but they're half of what they were before, and they're on half the meds they were on before—that is significant.

Even people who do keto dieting and don't want to fast, eating in a time-restricted window can help them lose a lot of weight. And intermittent fasting can be even more powerful because it's sustainable. Usually we recommend extended fasts for people in extreme situations of obesity, but people can't do the extended fasts for long periods of time. Intermittent fasting will fit into their life over the long term.

Q: *What are some of your favorite tips and tricks for fasting days?*

A: Don't think about fasting! We're rebellious by nature. If you think about the fact that you're fasting, all you're doing is thinking about not fasting. A recent patient told me that at 3 p.m. is her worst time when she's always hungry. I told to her to plan an activity at that time.

Q: *Do you do anything special to take care of yourself when you're fasting?*

A: Stay hydrated. Sometimes, depending on the individual, supplementing with electrolytes is important. Refeeding syndrome is important, but not a big risk because most of us trying to fast aren't malnourished—we're overnourished!

And just keep busy. Don't be a sedentary rock. Drink water to prevent against headaches and feeling nauseous from getting dehydrated during the fast. Especially if you have a lot of stored glycogen because your insulin levels are very high, you'll pee and lose a lot of water—usually the biggest drops are in the first three days—so you have to remember to hydrate. I used to set an alarm on my phone to drink a glass of water every 50 minutes, just to make sure I didn't forget.

Q: *What are the biggest mistakes you see people make when fasting?*

A: Trying to figure out what they can have on their fast. That and people obsessing over the fact that they're fasting. I think in the fasting and keto world, there's a lot of talk about stuff that's not necessarily required in terms of electrolytes. I just recommend not to focus so much on the fasting, and work on other behaviors and what you're going to do with your productivity. It's the moment people obsess with their fasting that they fail.

Also, really try to experiment and figure out what works for you. Just because something works for someone else doesn't mean it's going to work for you. Just because someone says online that they did a ten-day fast, doesn't mean you'll be able to do one. But if you do a 24-hour fast or a 36-hour fast three days a week, you'll get the same results.

Q: *Can you talk about the importance of varying your food intake—fasting and feasting?*

A: Well, you need to eat! You want to change things up day in and day out. When you eat, you give the body food energy—it's like a budget. The body allocates this much to the respiratory system, this much to the reproductive system, etc. When you're fasting, you're trying to create an energy deficit—you're pulling energy out of storage. When people eat the same amount every day, their body adapts to that budget, and the system slows down and they just stop losing weight.

When you're fasting, you throw your body off so the metabolic rate doesn't have time to adjust.

Q: *How can people learn more about IDM or work with you?*

A: You can subscribe on a monthly basis to the online membership community, which has a training course, interactive Q&A, and community support. Or, you can get online one-on-one coaching specific to your individual situation. You can find both at idmprogram.com.

Drink Enough Fluids

If you recall from Chapter 3, fasting depletes glycogen stores, and a lot of water is lost with the glycogen. This accounts for some weight loss and can also result in dehydration if you're not mindful of replenishing your fluids. This is doubly important if you're on a ketogenic diet, because you won't replenish glycogen or its associated water when you eat.

A lot of us are so busy that we don't pay much attention to drinking water throughout the day. Hydration is extremely important on a fast, and you can end up feeling really terrible if you forget to drink enough water on your fasting days. Carbonated water, also called seltzer, club soda, or sparkling water, is a great treat when fasting. It's a little more exciting than regular water, and it's a nice thing to order if you're out at a restaurant and don't want to eat or drink.

In addition to water and carbonated water, herbal tea is a great option when fasting. Herbal tea is made from the dried leaves of flowers and herbs, and doesn't have caffeine. It is hydrating, and you can drink as much as you like! Examples are chamomile, rooibos, lavender, mint, and dandelion root.

Be sure to read the ingredient list and avoid teas that include ground ingredients like cacao that contain calories, or those that include sweeteners. You can also drink caffeinated tea, but of course, you will feel the effects of the caffeine. Black tea, green tea, oolong, and fermented teas are all good to have, but, like coffee, you will have a tolerance limit for the caffeine and won't want to drink too much of it, or drink it at night. That's where the herbal teas come in handy!

Some people incorporate bone broth, such as chicken or beef broth, into their fasting regimen, especially if they are doing multi-day fasts and find it challenging to go without food entirely during that time. For very few calories (100 to 200 per bowl), they can drink some broth and feel rejuvenated. It is hydrating (good when you're fasting), provides minerals and electrolytes (it's good to salt your broth), and provides some amino acids as well. The smell and taste of the broth can relieve hunger. Of course, because broth does deliver nutrients to the body, it will trigger nutrient sensors that tell the body you are no longer fasting. A small rise in insulin should occur. This is a small effect relative to eating a meal, so it's not a total loss—and many people find that they are able to fast longer if they include broth in their fasting days, so the trade-off works out in the end. However, it doesn't make sense to have broth for fasts of a day or less since most people can go that long without eating and feel just fine—and the whole point of a fasting practice is to actually fast during your fasting time! Either way, broth is good to consume during your eating window to get the benefits of hydration and a dose of minerals.

Consume Sodium, Potassium, and Magnesium Regularly

Electrolytes are minerals that perform essential functions in the body, such as moving nutrients into and out of cells, supporting nerve impulses, and supporting muscle contractions, including those of the heart muscle. The function of these minerals is very well regulated in a healthy person. Sodium, potassium, and magnesium are all electrolytes. Their concentration depends a lot on the amount of water in the body, and therefore dehydration (or overhydration) can cause an imbalance of electrolytes.

You hear a lot about sodium in connection with fasting and ketogenic dieting because your kidneys excrete more sodium while you're fasting, and levels of potassium and magnesium can be affected too. The best way to ensure you have enough sodium, potassium, and magnesium is to consume these minerals in your diet. Contrary to conventional wisdom, do not be afraid of salt! There is good evidence to suggest that limiting sodium to about 2000 mg per day is not ideal and can be harmful. Sodium needs for someone who is fasting, or on a ketogenic diet, are much higher, between 3000 to 5000 mg per day. I generally discourage calculating nutrient intakes unless you are managing a health problem that requires nutrient monitoring (e.g., diabetes, kidney disease) or are using diet to enhance athletic performance and seeking a narrow range of intake. For the majority of us just trying to have a healthy diet and avoid weight gain, it's quite cumbersome to track how much sodium we consume every day! It's simplest to focus on adding salt to your diet. Put salt on your food and use it liberally when cooking. If you drink broth, salt your broth. If you eat avocados, cucumber slices, or tomato slices on their own, sprinkle salt on them! It's delicious, and will help you maintain a good sodium level.

Magnesium and potassium are found in varying amounts in nearly all types of whole foods. Focus your diet on vegetables, meat and fish, high-quality dairy, nuts, and some fruits. Nuts like almonds and cashews are rich in magnesium, as are avocados, green vegetables, salmon and other fish, and dairy products. Potassium is found in dark green leafy vegetables, dairy products, meat and fish, legumes like lentils and beans, winter squash, sweet potatoes, some nuts and seeds, and dried fruit.

Most adults in the United States consume less magnesium and less potassium than is recommended. Magnesium deficiency can cause fatigue, weakness, and muscle cramps. If you notice these symptoms, you can take a magnesium supplement of up to 400 mg per day. Potassium deficiency can cause similar symptoms of muscle cramps and twitching, as well as irregular heart rate. Potassium supplements are not very common, as taking too much can be dangerous. It's best to eat a diet rich in the foods mentioned.

If you're only fasting for periods of a day or less and eating mineral-rich foods on your eating days, then it's not likely you will have a problem with electrolytes. If you are fasting in combination with a ketogenic diet, then you may have to pay closer attention and look out for symptoms of electrolyte imbalance.

Break Your Fast with Something Small

It's a good idea to eat a small meal or snack to break your fast, and see whether you have the appetite for a full meal. You don't have to eat any special foods, but you simply may not have room for much right away. If you're fasting for a day or less, there's no harm to breaking your fast with a typical meal if that's what works in your schedule—you just may notice that you can't finish it, and choose to put the rest away for later.

If you're fasting for a couple of days, then it's more important to go slowly when you start to eat again. Have something light that's not too hard on the digestive tract. A common tradition for breaking the fast of Ramadan is to eat one date, the sugary fruit of the date palm that you may know better in its dried version. This small dose of sugar gets digestive juices flowing and prepares the body to receive more food. I am not exactly a fan of sugary things, so I prefer to have just a few bites of a meal and wait a while until I've grown an appetite for the rest. You might want to break your fast with a small cup of broth-based soup (cream-based is tougher on the digestive tract), a small green salad, or something else that you know agrees with you. I recommend avoiding fried foods, very acidic foods (like tomato sauce or orange juice), large amounts of sugar or flour (e.g., cake, cookies, pasta), and dairy products, as these tend to cause bloating and upset stomach if eaten after a period of fasting.

Cut Down on Your Alcohol Consumption

If you do drink alcohol, give some thought to how and whether you want to modify your drinking habits to accommodate your new fasting habit. (If you're not a drinker, good for you! That's one less thing to tackle.) I notice that folks who drink seem to be in two camps when it comes to modifying their drinking patterns to start an intermittent fasting practice. On the one hand, there are those who want to cut out drinking entirely as part of their new diet habits. They'll have it easier when they start fasting, and depending on the amount they drink, will likely lose more weight without the alcohol. The other group doesn't want to cut out drinking, but may cut down in amount or frequency. They'll have to do a bit more scheduling work, because alcohol can make fasting a bit trickier.

Know that alcohol will affect your appetite in unpredictable ways, both on the day you're drinking, and the day after. So if you drink alcohol at night and expect to fast the next day, you may be in for an unpleasant fast. Alcohol is dehydrating, and fasting is too, so you'll need even more fluid on your fast. If drinking alcohol makes you to want to binge on starchy foods, well, you may just be playing with fire there. These are just considerations for you. Use common sense about how drinking will affect your fasting practice, and make adjustments that help you achieve the goals that matter to you. Alcohol is by no means "banned." If you're someone who is disciplined with drinking and your alcohol consumption consists of one glass of wine or a cocktail at dinner, you'll be able to gauge how the drink affects your fast and figure out the best way to work around it. If you drink more heavily, then you may want to consider cutting down.

Take Time to Adjust

Fasting increases adrenaline levels, readying the body for action. That's because fasting, like exercise, is a mild form of stress that results in some positive changes in the body. While fasting, noradrenaline helps the body focus strength and resources on getting through the "challenge"—that is, it gives you energy and mental focus to go out and find food. Remember, the body's hormonal system doesn't know we have grocery stores now; it thinks we still have to go out and hunt animals for food! So adrenaline increases your heart and metabolic rates, and releases stored glucose and fat into the bloodstream to provide energy for the hunt. This is, of course, very good for weight loss, but it's *not* always good for sleeping.

If, during your fasting window, you find that you're jittery, have trouble falling asleep, or wake up abruptly in the middle of the night, it's likely that adrenaline is the culprit. Take steps to minimize the impact of this hormone on your schedule. You may want to quit drinking caffeine for a while, and practice sleep meditation or take a nightly bath to put you in a calm mood before bed. Take advantage of the extra energy and focus to be more productive and tackle tasks that have been on your to-do list for a while, even if that means knocking them out at odd hours of the night. And remember—adrenaline is keeping your metabolic rate high, and your body burning through more fat. Hopefully that's motivation enough to make it through the energy highs if they're bothersome to you.

Don't Start Fasting in Periods of High Stress

You're probably familiar with the hormone cortisol. Cortisol, like adrenaline, is produced in the body as a response to stress and is meant to help focus the body's faculties on overcoming the stress and returning to normal. The relevant difference is that cortisol levels can remain high over a long period of time if the body is under chronic stress. One of cortisol's main functions is to trigger the release of glucose into the blood. Insulin levels rise in response. In a momentarily stressful situation, this system would provide the body with energy needed to fight or flee whatever stressor it faced. But persistently elevated cortisol levels can keep blood sugar and insulin levels persistently high and lead to weight gain and insulin resistance. If you are in a period of high stress in your life—whether because of a job change, relationship troubles, an illness, or other difficult time—then it's probably not the best time to start your fast. If you're eager to get started anyway, then keep to the time-restricted eating approach (fast for 16 hours and eat within an 8-hour window every day) and avoid longer fasts until the stress has subsided.

Exercise on Empty

I get asked all the time if it's okay to work out "on an empty stomach." The answer is yes! It is safe and perfectly normal for the average person to do some exercise without having had any food. In general, a healthy adult will not have adverse reactions to exercising on an empty stomach. If you're seeking weight loss, then working out without eating will help you burn through fat more quickly—even more so if you've already done an overnight fast. Plus, as we discussed above, adrenaline levels are higher when you fast, so you'll likely have more energy to commit to your exercise routine if you choose to exercise fasted.

That said, if you are someone who has a history of feeling weak, faint, or dizzy after exercise on an empty stomach, and you know that it's not the right thing for you, then don't do it. Pay attention to your body, and don't do something that makes you feel bad. If fasted workouts don't suit you, it's certainly wise to arrange an exercise schedule that fits with your fasting schedule in a way that allows you to feel good while doing both. One of the great things about fasting, as I've said before, is you can pretty much arrange it how you like. Just pick a time to fast that doesn't conflict with the training you want to do.

For the rest of us, exercising on empty is a nice hack that can speed fat loss. I would hate for you to miss out on it because you've been taught that you'll become dangerously hypoglycemic if you don't have a pre-workout, carb-based snack. Consider this: many adults all over the world perform some type of manual labor in the course of their day just to make a living, get around, or provide sustenance for their families. Many communities in Africa, Asia, and South America practice subsistence farming and walk long distances to get basic necessities like water and cooking fuel. And many of them do this without obsessing over what to eat before their "workout." The human body is not as fragile as you may think!

Risks of Fasting

When thinking of the potential risks of fasting, I am drawn to share an excerpt from a paper titled "Fasting for Weight Loss: An Effective Strategy or Lasting Dieting Trend?" published in the *International Journal of Obesity* in 2015. It compares the potential risks of fasting to those of gastric bypass surgery, in which a portion of the stomach is cut out to reduce the amount of food a person can consume, thereby reducing their weight. It says: "Although there is some long-term success with gastric surgical operations for morbid obesity, there is still a requirement for dietary approaches for weight management… particularly as invasive interventions carry post-operative risk of death due to complications." What they're saying is that although cutting out a part of a person's stomach can make them eat less, the surgery might also kill them. To me, it is quite sad that we are willing to go to such lengths to force weight loss instead of simply recommending fasting as a way to dramatically lose extra fat. I would hope that it's easy to see that skipping meals sometimes, or even going without food for a day or two—which many people around the world do—is simply not in a category of risk anywhere near on par with that of surgery to remove part of a major organ.

There are very few risks of fasting for someone who is well-nourished to begin with. The scariest thing you will hear of in connection with risks of fasting is "refeeding syndrome," but it is not a realistic concern for any healthy, well-nourished person practicing intermittent fasting in the short periods described in this book. Refeeding syndrome is a very dangerous and potentially deadly condition of electrolyte and fluid imbalance that may occur when malnourished people, such as those with severe anorexia or people who have been hospitalized for a long time, begin eating again after a long period of no food intake. It is seen most often in hospitalized individuals being fed through a feeding tube, and dietitians in the hospital will calculate a safe concentration of nutrients and electrolytes to administer to patients upon refeeding to prevent this complication. Having a very low body weight and not eating for more than 10 days significantly increases the risk of refeeding syndrome. That's why fasting is not recommended for someone who is underweight or poorly nourished, deficient in any nutrients (e.g., anemic), and why fasts longer than a few days are not recommended without medical supervision.

If you're practicing multi-day fasts without medical supervision, keep your fasts under five days, and make sure to eat a nourishing diet when you're not fasting. If you want to try fasts longer than those described in this book, find a healthcare professional who can provide you more customized support and supervision. Similarly, if you adopt an intermittent fasting lifestyle and choose not to eat a healthful diet on your eating days, you could be at increased risk for nutrient deficiencies, including deficiencies for vitamins, minerals, and essential fatty acids. Even if you don't practice fasting, you will be at risk if you eat a poor-quality diet. The simple solution to this is to eat well during your eating window. We'll discuss how to eat well in Chapter 9.

As mentioned, fasting can be dehydrating, so be sure to drink lots of fluids and replace your electrolytes, especially if you're sweating or exercising a lot. Another risk of fasting is that it may take you away from social activities that are a source of enjoyment for you if those activities center around food and drink (and you choose not to participate while fasting). In that case, it's smart to fill your calendar with other activities that better support your fasting habit, such as meeting up with friends for a walk or bike ride, taking a class, practicing a new hobby, or going to local events. Finally, it's important to nurture habits that make you feel nourished and soothed that don't involve eating or drinking. Many of us turn to foods like ice cream or other "comfort foods" when feeling down, or go out for a drink to relax after a long work week. These habits can get in the way of a successful fast! Explore some other self-soothing practices such as taking a bath, writing in a journal, or calling a friend when you need some support. Make it a point to practice self-care in ways that don't include eating or drinking.

Lastly, there are some discomforts you may experience when beginning to fast. You may be hungry sometimes when you are fasting, or fear being hungry even when you're not. The hormone ghrelin contributes to the physiological part of hunger, and it comes and goes in waves, as discussed in Chapter 4. Keeping busy helps get you through a ghrelin peak. Most people find the psychological barrier to fasting is the more difficult one to overcome, especially in the beginning. To that, I again suggest finding a buddy or a community of people who fast to demystify the unknown and stop ruminating on it. Additionally, Some people feel irritable the first few times they skip a meal because they are not used to doing so. People who are very dependent on carbs may go through a transition period of feeling lethargic or just plain bad the first few times they fast, though you can lessen the likelihood of that by reducing your carb intake and increasing your fat intake now, shifting toward a high-fat, very low-carb diet. The better able your cells are the use fat for energy, the easier fasting will be.

If you want more tips for taking care of yourself on your fast, check out my 15 Tips to Help You Succeed on an Intermittent Fast, downloadable at kristenmancinelli.com/15-tips-succeed-on-intermittent-fast.

CHAPTER 9

How to Eat When It's Time to Eat

Intermittent fasting is only half the fun. The other half is intermittent eating! And when you eat, you must eat well. On your eating days, eat to satisfaction! I often see people get so excited about their progress and the fact that they're able to go a whole day without eating that they think to themselves, "Oh, I'll just go light on this meal," and the next meal, and the next. Or they avoid fat when they eat because it's calorie dense and they think that keeping calories low all the time will speed their weight loss. Or they find some other strategy that amounts to alternating bouts of fasting with bouts of calorie-restricted eating. This is a mistake! This approach will result in the dreaded slowdown of metabolism that causes weight plateau and regain. Instead, focus on getting a wide variation in energy intake—from no energy one day while you're fasting, to lots of energy the next day while you're eating.

I'm not going to dive into a big explanation of why you should eat mostly whole, unprocessed foods. Collectively, we are very aware that the average American diet based on processed foods and lots of sugar is making us fat and sick. If you've read this far into a book about how to lose weight and improve your health, then you're already highly motivated to jump off that bandwagon. It's especially important to eat a robustly nutritious diet when you practice intermittent fasting because you have to get all your nourishment in a shorter window of time. To do this, eat what you want, as long as what you're eating has been grown on trees, from the ground, or in the seabed, or was once a living animal, and hasn't been altered much on its way to your plate. Whatever you're eating, put salt on it. Most people would benefit from eating more fat and fewer carbs. Don't overdo the protein. Avoid processed and packaged foods at all costs. And don't eat anything cooked in "vegetable oil."

Eat a Good Amount of Fat

Fat is satiating, so you stay full longer after a meal with fat than one without it. Fat doesn't increase insulin levels, so it won't contribute to insulin resistance the ways carbs will. If you've struggled with weight loss on a low-fat diet in the past, or you have poor discipline when it comes to carbohydrates, then focus on getting more fat and pushing some of the carbs off your plate. There are different types of fats, and optimal health is achieved by eating a variety of fats. Here's a quick review:

Monounsaturated fats are found in high amounts in avocados and olives and their oils, and most nuts and seeds. These fats are a cornerstone of the Mediterranean diet and are linked to lower risk of heart disease. As a rule of thumb, it's good to eat more monounsaturated fat.

Saturated fats are found in fatty portions of foods from land animals, such as the skin of a chicken, the marbling of a steak, or the extra fat in bacon or pork belly. Butter and dairy products are also high in saturated fat. The only plant foods rich in saturated fat are coconut and palm oils. Saturated fat has long been demonized because it was believed to be a major cause of heart disease, but that theory has not proved true. There is no reason to avoid saturated fat. However, many people fail to consume other types of fat and get most of their fat in the form of saturated fat, which isn't ideal. It's important to vary your fat intake. So if you tell me you don't like fish or avocado and just want to get all your fat from bacon and steak, I'll tell you to be a little more open minded. Try some new things! There are lots of recipes in Chapter 10 to help you out.

Polyunsaturated fats are found in plant foods and fish, and there are two types that are important to differentiate: omega-3 fats, which most people need to consume more of, and omega-6 fats, which practically everyone needs to consume less of. The balance of omega-3 and omega-6 fats is extremely important for overall health, and excess omega-6 fats contribute to inflammation and diseases associated with it, including obesity, diabetes, and cardiovascular disease.

Food sources of omega-3 fats are rare, which is why we struggle to get enough of them. The active forms of omega-3 fats are eicosapentaenoic acid (EPA) and docosahexaenoic acid (DHA) found mainly in fatty fish like salmon, mackerel, and herring, and in smaller amounts in tuna and other commonly eaten fish, including shellfish. If you don't eat those foods, you're likely not getting very much of the active forms of omega-3 fats. Flaxseed, chia seeds, and walnuts contain a good amount of omega-3 fats but not in the active form, and conversion inside the body is minimal—so it's important to get the fat from seafood sources directly.

Omega-6 fats are found in almost all processed foods and foods prepared outside the home. They are the main fat type found in seed oils such as soybean, corn, or vegetable oil that are cheap and ubiquitous in North America—so unless we make a real effort to avoid these fats, we eat them almost constantly. This is not good for metabolic health. The negative impact of omega-6 fats is even worse when omega-3 intake is low. The takeaway is to avoid low-quality seed oils, cook with olive or coconut oil, and eat more fatty fish!

Incorporating Fat into Your Diet

I recommend cooking everything in olive oil unless you're looking for a specific flavor from butter, animal fat, or coconut oil. There's a misguided belief that olive oil should only be used for cold preparations because it doesn't have a high smoke point, but it's perfectly okay to use olive oil for baking, roasting, or sautéing foods. I wouldn't use olive oil for frying, but then again, I wouldn't recommend frying your food. Use olive oil for salad dressings, as well. Drizzle olive oil on top of any finished meal that's light on fat.

Eat avocados. Avocados are a uniquely high-fat, nutrient-rich fruit, and I recommend you make them a regular part of your diet. If you live in a part of the world where avocados are not easy to get in the regular supermarket, visit a Latin American grocery store in your vicinity. There, you will find avocados, most likely ripe and reasonably priced. You can buy a few at a time and leave them in the fridge if they are close to ripe or out on the counter for a couple of days if they're not. Eat avocados sliced on the side of your meal, or make avocado mash or guacamole regularly. Use avocados in sauces or dressings to thicken them. If you're really not a fan of avocados, include avocado oil in your diet. Both avocados and olives (as well as their oils) are high in monounsaturated fat that most people would benefit from eating more of.

Use liberal amounts of olive, avocado, and coconut oil or butter in your cooking. Fat transfers heat from the pan to the food, allowing for well-rounded cooking. Fat also carries flavor and adds moisture to a dish—you will notice a *significant* difference in flavor when you use a good amount of oil to sauté leafy greens, for instance, rather than just enough oil to coat the bottom of the pan. Don't be afraid to use a lot of fat when cooking! This is the secret to flavor in restaurant dishes, because chefs are not afraid of fat at all. Don't just leave a piece of meat or a portion of vegetables naked on your plate. Finish dishes with fat-rich sauces or dressings like tahini or cream sauce, or oil-based condiments like pesto or chimichurri.

There are other simple ways to get more fat in your diet. If you eat dairy products like yogurt and cheese, always choose the full-fat version. Always eat whole eggs rather than just egg whites. Swap out grain flours, such as wheat, for nut flours, such as almond, in baking recipes. Include a handful of nuts before or after a meal that doesn't contain a lot of fat. Use full-fat, pure coconut milk instead of dairy milk or processed nut or grain milks (e.g., almond, oat) in smoothies, curries, or any desserts you make.

Eat Protein in Moderation

More is not necessarily better when it comes to protein. The average person in the United States consumes more protein than needed to meet their needs. We are accustomed to a large piece of meat on our plate—usually with a double serving of starch and a stingy portion of vegetables. This is a distorted view of what a meal should be. Aim for a little less meat, way less starch, and more green vegetables (unless you're on a ketogenic diet, which we'll discuss below).

Lean toward fattier cuts of meats so you can achieve higher fat intake. Eat the dark meat and the skin of the chicken rather than just a breast—and no skinless breasts, please! Select marbled cuts of beef such as rib eye over lean cuts like sirloin, and talk to the butcher to get more familiar with the fat content of the cuts available at your grocer. Look for ground beef with an 80/20 ratio of lean meat to fat rather than a 90/10 ratio. Opt for lamb instead of beef when you can find it. Choose fatty fish like salmon and mackerel over lean fish like sole/flounder, tilapia, or cod, and eat the skin of the fish too. Enjoy bacon and pork belly instead of leaner cuts like pork tenderloin or pork chop. If you like organ meats like heart, liver, and other innards, eat those for their high fat and/or high mineral content. Broth made from the bones of beef, chicken, or other animal is a good source of the minerals that are important during fasting, and also provides some protein and a small amount of fat.

Eggs and dairy products also provide some protein, as do nuts and seeds. Legumes such as lentils, black beans, or chickpeas are good vegan protein sources.

Eat Non-Starchy Vegetables

Since you're fasting to lower insulin levels and allow fat burning to happen, it's not a great idea to eat a lot of carb-heavy foods like bread, potatoes, rice, sweet potatoes, or other starches, or to consume sugary foods like desserts or sweetened beverages (including sugar in your tea or coffee). That will just result in high blood sugar, followed by high insulin levels and renewed hunger when blood sugar falls back down. You'll eat again—and mostly carbs—soon after you've digested your meal, triggering another round of high insulin and quickly renewed hunger. This is the cycle that leads to insulin resistance and weight gain in the first place!

It's better to eat fewer carbs, and more nutritious ones, which you can do by focusing on non-starchy vegetables along with small amounts of starches and fruit (though, if you're eating a ketogenic diet, you won't consume starch or fruit at all). These foods contribute fiber, water, and vitamins and minerals to your diet, all essential to supporting weight loss and maintaining good health.

Eat lots of leafy greens like spinach, arugula, salad greens, mustard greens, bok choy, and kale. Eat other brassicas like broccoli, Brussels sprouts, cabbage, and cauliflower. Think of cucumber slices or blanched asparagus spears instead of chips or bread when you need something to dip into, say, guacamole or hummus. Wild mushrooms are an excellent addition to most people's diets, as they are low in calories and high in lots of micronutrients, plus they're delicious and have a "meaty" or umami flavor when cooked. Sea vegetables like algae are highly nutritious and often forgotten about in our culture. If you're not familiar, try a seaweed salad the next time you're at a restaurant that serves one, as you may find you like it! You can also add spirulina, a powdered form of seaweed, to smoothies. Use alliums like garlic and onion; roots like ginger, turmeric, and horseradish; and herbs like basil, cilantro, thyme and rosemary in your cooking, as these plant foods have great medicinal properties and add layers of flavor to your food.

Eat Fermented and Vinegared Foods

Fermented vegetables like kimchi and sauerkraut are becoming popular these days thanks to an increased understanding of their health benefits. The live bacteria living in these and other fermented foods take up residence in our digestive tracts and contribute to overall good health. Fermented foods are made by allowing bacteria to consume the sugar or starch in the original raw products, turning it into acid and giving the end product a sour flavor. Yogurt, miso (the fermented soybean paste used in miso soup), and sourdough bread are all examples of fermented foods. Nowadays, due to their popularity, you can find lots of fermented vegetables in health-focused grocery stores. I like to add these to my plate to give a nice flavor kick to meat or eggs.

Non-fermented pickles are also a great addition to the diet. These are made simply by putting raw vegetables into a salt-and-vinegar solution. What you get is the common cucumber pickle that often comes on the side of your sandwich. Commercial pickle products tend to have sugar and synthetic preservatives added to them, and I wouldn't choose those. But many grocery stores will have local brands of higher-quality pickles to choose from. And it's not just cucumbers that can be pickled—you can pickle cauliflower, onions, okra, and pretty much anything you want! Of course you can pickle your own vegetables, and there are some recipes in Chapter 10. Pickling vegetables lowers their carbohydrate content and preserves them for eating when fresh vegetables are not in season (which is important if you live in a seasonal climate).

Foods to Avoid

In general, don't eat any food that your great-great-grandmother wouldn't recognize as food. Another rule of thumb is to make sure the food hasn't been changed much from its original form, and that the original is recognizable in the final product. Take apple juice as an example. Looking at a glass of apple juice, can you tell it came from an apple? Not really, so I wouldn't consume it. What about canned whole tomatoes? They look pretty much like raw tomatoes, only they're cooked. They pass the test. An exception to this rule is olive and coconut oils, which don't look like olives or coconuts at all! These foods are good to eat, and you should look for the word "virgin" on the label to make sure they're not processed more than necessary.

Avoid Processed Foods

I don't eat or recommend that others eat processed foods—yes, technically, fermented vegetables and cured meats are processed foods because of the methods used to transform them from their raw, natural states into their final form, but that's not what I'm talking about here. When I say processed foods, I mean things in a box or package with a Nutrition Facts panel on them. Cereal, crackers, microwavable mac and cheese, frozen burritos, and jarred sauces made thick with xanthan gum are examples of the types of foods I am talking about. For simplicity's sake, I'll refer to these types of processed foods as "junk food."

I'll give a special mention here to "bars." Do not eat "bars." Food bars, energy bars, breakfast bars, meal replacement bars, whatever-you-want-to-call-them-bars—avoid these at all costs. Bars are just amalgamations of some sugar (agave nectar, date paste, evaporated cane juice, or sugar by some other fancy name) smushed together with some nuts or seeds and sprinkled with protein powder. They honestly remind me of the concentrated food pellets used to fatten up mice in the biochemistry lab I worked in after college. You, a human being, should eat real food. Please.

Your appetite for having real, nourishing food over junk food is improved when you fast. Once you go half a day or more without eating, when the time comes, you are ready for something wholesome. That said, if you eat a junk food diet despite this, intermittent fasting will probably help mitigate the effects of your poor food choices on your health. So if you are unable or unwilling to cut out these foods, then at a minimum, you should incorporate an intermittent fasting practice into your life.

Avoid Seed Oils

Seed oils are oils extracted from the seed of any plant as opposed to its fruit. Earlier, I recommended using olive, avocado, or coconut. These oils are produced from the fruit of the tree and produce healthy oils with a beneficial nutrient profile. In contrast, seed oils are produced from plant seeds such as soybeans, cottonseed, or corn kernels, and are much too high in inflammatory omega-6 fats. "Vegetable oil" is usually a mixture of these and is an equally bad choice. Moreover, these oils are industrially produced (i.e., you can't make them in your home kitchen), and that extra processing does not work in our favor when it comes to dietary health. Finally, these oils are extremely cheap and don't spoil very easily—making them an excellent choice for use in prepared and processed food products that are optimized for cheap production and long shelf-life.

You probably consume a lot of seed oils if you often eat out at restaurants or eat packaged foods. It's best to eliminate unnecessary sources of seed oils from your diet. When eating out, ask about the types of oils they use in the kitchen, and steer toward those that use olive oil, butter, or animal fats. If you have bottles of vegetable oil in your home, toss them now.

Avoid Alcohol

Alcohol obviously isn't a category of food. I've included it here because alcohol contains calories, which means it provides energy and can promote weight gain just like other calorie-containing ingestibles. Many people believe that the calories in alcoholic beverages come solely from sweeteners and juice-based mixers added to them. That's not true. Alcohol provides 7 cal per gram all on its own. Any juice, sugar, or syrup added to the drink will tack on additional calories in the form of carbohydrates. Drinks made with egg white will also have protein calories, while those made with cream will additional have fat calories.

The internet would have you believe that certain spirit alcohols, such as vodka or gin, are calorie-free or "not as fattening" as other spirits—or, my personal favorite, that vodka and other colorless spirits have fewer carbs than whiskey, rum, and other amber-colored ones. Let's set the record straight once and for all: distilled spirits do not contain carbohydrates in any amount whatsoever. Zero. No carbs. No fat or protein, either. That's because spirits are produced in a process called distillation, in which a fermented mash of carbohydrate is heated so that the liquid (ethanol) boils and becomes a gas, travels through a tube, cools, transforms back into a liquid and settles into a new container. The mash containing all the carbohydrate is left behind in the old container. You might remember this process from high school chemistry class where you separated salt or another dissolved solid from the liquid in which it was dissolved. It seemed like magic at the time, but now it's just booze (which some might say is magic, too).

Wine and beer are different from distilled spirits in that they do contain some residual carbohydrate from their respective starting products (grapes in the case of wine, and grains in the case of beer). That's because wine and beer are mechanically separated (e.g., filtered) from their starting products and do not go through a distillation process. Below is a chart of average calorie counts and carbohydrate content for common alcoholic beverages.

Average Calories per Alcoholic Beverage

Beverage	Serving size	Calories from carbohydrates per serving	Calories from alcohol per serving	Total calories per serving
Gin, vodka, rum, whiskey (80 proof)	1.5 fl. oz.	0 cal	97 cal	97 cal
White wine	5 fl. oz.	16 cal	105 cal	121 cal
Red wine	5 fl. oz.	16 cal	109 cal	125 cal
Rose wine	5 fl. oz.	24 cal	122 cal	126 cal
Beer	12 fl. oz.	50 cal	100 cal	150 cal

Source: USDA National Nutrient Database for Standard Reference

You should know that alcohol may interfere with your fast in various ways and I wholeheartedly discourage it. For one thing, your liver will prioritize metabolizing alcohol to get it out of your system. It will do so at the expense of other important processes, including breaking down fatty acids for energy and stimulating gluconeogenesis—the key metabolic processes you're trying to promote when fasting! I came across a striking example of this in a paper titled "Ethanol Causes Acute Inhibition of Carbohydrate, Fat, and Protein Oxidation and Insulin Resistance" in the *Journal of Clinical Investigation,* where ethanol infusion caused an 87 percent decrease in fat oxidation. Energy contributions from fat dropped from 70 percent to about 10 percent, and the remaining 60 percent of energy needs were met with the ethanol itself. Similar effects are seen on glucose use for energy needs. In other words, alcohol consumption will shut down fat, protein, and glucose oxidation, and will then meet most of the body's energy needs until it is eliminated. If you drink alcohol, you won't get back to burning fat until it's all used up.

The Ketogenic Diet and Fasting

It's no secret that I'm a fan of both the lower-than-average and very-low-carb/ketogenic approaches. I think the very-low-carb approach brings tremendous benefits to many people, and it's gotten a bad rap for far too long. It might be fun to try if you're already an experienced faster.

That said, don't feel you have to go keto if it really doesn't appeal to you. Some people have dietary preferences that make keto unfeasible (vegans, for example, would have a very hard time meeting their nutrient needs on a ketogenic diet). But let's be very clear: there is no "kind of" keto or "halfway" keto. You're either on a ketogenic diet or you're not. If you're not, then you're on a low-carb diet, and you'll likely have better weight loss results than anyone on a moderate- or high-carb diet. If you're going keto, then there are some points to review.

What a Ketogenic Diet Is Not

I generally like to focus on what a dietary strategy *is* and how it works to promote weight loss and prevent disease. I avoid harping on what you can't eat or defining a diet by explaining how it's different than something else. But after countless conversations with individuals who believe they are on a ketogenic diet when they are not, and after reading numerous articles on "how to go keto!" that don't quite capture it, I've decided to take a different approach. The following dietary strategies are not equivalent to a ketogenic diet.

Low-carb is not necessarily keto. On a low-carb diet, you'll avoid foods that we consider starchy or sugary. You won't eat sweets like desserts, pastries, muffins, cookies, candy, or chocolate, or any dried fruits like dried mango, raisins, or others. You won't consume sugary beverages like soda, juice, sweetened tea or coffee, cold-pressed juices, or electrolyte replacement drinks such as Gatorade. You won't eat foods made with grain flour, such as breads, pasta, crackers, or any whole grain foods, including rice, quinoa, couscous, farro, etc. You may also eliminate potatoes and other starchy vegetables including sweet potatoes, winter squash, and corn. You *will* eat lots of non-starchy vegetables—as much as you want! However, you will *not* eat unlimited non-starchy vegetables if you're following a ketogenic diet.

High fat is not necessarily keto. Eating lots of fat while also eating lots of carbs is not only not keto, it's terrible for your health. Adding MCT oil to your normal diet does not make you "a keto warrior." Just upping your fat intake—even artificially increasing your blood ketone levels—does not mean you're ketogenic. The genesis part of the word "ketogenic" implies that your body is *generating* the ketones from your body fat.

High protein is definitely not keto. It's hard to believe that this is still a point of confusion, but it is. A ketogenic diet is one in which your protein intake is low to moderate. It's not a meat-based diet. To do keto properly, you will need to eat smaller portions of meat and focus on fattier cuts—no lean proteins, no egg whites, no skinless chicken breasts.

Cleaning up your diet by eliminating sugary, processed foods is far from keto. You have to make much more dramatic changes than that. Additionally, eating lots of keto junk foods like fat bombs and "keto cake" may technically fit into a ketogenic diet, but I don't recommend it! Aim to eat real food. If it can't be made delicious without a synthetic sweetener like erythritol, it's probably not worth eating.

What Is a Ketogenic Diet?

A ketogenic diet is any diet in which the body is producing ketones at a level high enough to contribute meaningfully to the body's energy needs. This really only happens when your carb intake is exceptionally low, protein intake is low to moderate, and fat intake is extremely high. (Of course, ketones also contribute significantly to energy needs during fasting, but fasting isn't considered a diet so much as it is a break from your diet.) On a ketogenic diet, your macronutrient ratios will be somewhere in the realm of 80 percent calories from fat, 15 percent from protein, and 5 percent from carbs. Another way of approaching the diet is to limit net carbs (total carbs minus fiber) to roughly 20 to 25 grams per day, eat 1 gram of protein per kilogram of body weight, and take the rest of your energy as fat.

The two biggest mistakes I see people make when attempting a ketogenic diet are eating too many vegetables and not eating enough fat. What many people seem to misunderstand is that you can't eat all the vegetables you want on a ketogenic diet! You can only have vegetables in very small amounts. This goes counter to everything we think we know about how to eat healthy and lose weight, so most people keep eating lots of vegetables, and they never achieve a ketogenic state!

Vegetables have carbs. Yes—kale, broccoli, and cucumbers all have carbs. Overall, the amount is very small. But you are only permitted a tiny allotment of carbs when you're on a ketogenic diet, so, you can't eat very many vegetables and stay in ketosis. Sure, if you're a keto-adapted athlete, a large man with a lot of lean body mass and a fast metabolism, or you're someone who's been properly intermittent fasting and ketogenic dieting for years, then you can probably get away with eating more vegetables and stay in ketosis or quickly bounce back without much trouble. But I'm guessing if you're reading this book, then you're not one of those super keto-adapted people, so you would have to limit your vegetable intake if you wanted to follow a ketogenic diet.

You also can't eat a lot of protein. Don't have 10-ounce steaks or four chicken thighs at every meal. Protein interferes with ketosis.

So what is left to eat? Fat. Not fat and lots of other stuff that we think of as diet foods, like chicken breast and extra-large kale salads. Just fat. This is hard to comprehend, because we don't eat anything that's pure fat. We don't eat sticks of butter, or spoonfuls of olive oil, or a nice cup of lard. So we really have a hard time wrapping our heads around this concept of a ketogenic diet. But it's quite doable if you are open-minded enough to try it. If so, I recommend you get a book on ketogenic dieting and explore it properly. My first book, *The Ketogenic Diet: A Scientifically Proven Approach to Fast, Healthy Weight Loss*, is focused entirely on how to follow a ketogenic diet and why it works to speed weight loss.

Breaking Your Fast

Some of my favorite eating moments happen when I'm fasting, and I wouldn't be doing a complete job if I didn't share some of my favorite meals with you. Breaking my fast is something of an occasion, and I participate more fully in the experience of eating. I don't gorge or get greedy when I eat. I just *appreciate* food more.

Since there are no specific food restrictions with fasting, I'm going to focus on the other major challenge many of us have to eating well: time. I'll walk you through how to prepare dozens of basic meals made from whole foods that are delicious and a lot less labor intensive than you might think. The focus will be on *technique*, which is the basis of all good cooking. If you master a few techniques—roasting vegetables, roasting meats, making emulsions or sauces, making stock—then a world of great meals will be open to you.

More than half of recipes that follow are for meals I typically eat, and they are not hard to make. The rest are more complex, for the adventurous among you! I am the first to confess that I am super lazy in the kitchen most of the time. Don't get me wrong—I love to cook when the mood is right. If it's a special occasion that calls for a big meal, like Thanksgiving or a visit from friends who live abroad, then I'll happily spend a few days preparing for the big feast and all day cooking it. If I've recently learned a new technique, like pickling vegetables, I will come home with 17 pounds of produce and enlist the help of friends to turn them into mouth-puckering delights in 32 mason jars that take up two shelves of my fridge for an entire year. In other words, I can really geek out on cooking and food prep when I want to.

However, I am *not* up for complicated, time-consuming cooking on any given night—especially when my eating window is about to close in one hour. It is very stressful to get home from work and realize you need to eat ASAP, and then set about creating a delicious meal from scratch. It's best to think ahead. So, here are the five cooking rules that get me through life without ever having to order take-out:

1. Whenever you cook, make enough for at least three meals, if not more. Freeze what you can't eat soon.

If you've ever made a soup, stew, or casserole (or even a pie, cake, or loaf of bread), you're inherently familiar with the concept of "batch cooking." You invest the time to make a pot of soup just once and know it'll feed you four or five times that week. You don't make one serving of soup from scratch each night for dinner. That would be a waste of time and energy.

Other foods can be batch cooked, too. I often roast a whole chicken, sear off two or three steaks at a time, make an egg frittata in a single pan that can last all week, and sauté three bunches of kale at once. The time saved is significant. For instance, just to prepare the kale, I use four kitchen tools: a cutting board and knife to chop the garlic, and a sauté pan and tongs to cook the kale; these all have to be washed after use, which can be one time if you batch cook, but five or six times if you cook one serving at a time.

The batch cooking method works very well for garnishes and condiments that can hold for months, such as preserved lemons, pickled onions, and pesto (freeze it). When your meal calls for a kick, you'll have a few flavor enhancers to choose from!

2. Use the scraps or leftovers of one meal for another.

Our grandmothers didn't throw away chicken carcasses, and neither should we! Instead, we should use them to make a tasty broth for our next soup. Store them in a sturdy zip-top plastic bag in the freezer until you get a few, and spend one day making a few quarts of broth to pull out as needed. You can do the same with lobster bodies and shrimp peels for a seafood broth, and the unwanted ends of vegetables for a vegetable broth.

When you fry bacon or other fatty meat, collect and strain the fat from the pan and store it in a glass jar in the fridge. You can use the fat when a dish would benefit from a meatier flavor than olive or coconut oil can offer (I like to put bacon fat in a bean casserole, for instance). Be sure to label the jars with a "P" for pork, "L" for lamb, and so on, or you'll go crazy trying to sort them out.

And when you get to that moment there are only two bites of a meal left, stop eating. Put the two bites back in their container in the fridge. You may want to make an omelet the next day, and that small amount of leftovers might just be a nice addition. Or you might end up throwing them out. It's okay.

3. Master the preparation of seven to ten meals.

It should be obvious that if you make a meal more than a dozen times, you'll get pretty good at it after a while and it will be easier than it was in the beginning. I find that many home cooks are sometimes too ambitious with their meal prep, trying new dishes on a weeknight from recipes they find on the web. This introduces the challenge of novelty into their food prep and could lead to more time spent, and more stress, than they'd planned for. Unless you are a seasoned cook and really love being in the kitchen, I strongly encourage you to keep it simple. Find a handful of meals that you like, and learn to make them well. Experiment with new dishes when you have lots of time to spare, and keep some leftovers on hand just in case.

4. Simplify recipes that seem too complicated.

I rarely follow recipes because they overwhelm me. They tend to include small amounts of lots of different things, and then I have to go buy those things, use them once, and let them go bad in the fridge later that week. Plus, I get tired of measuring and chopping all those different ingredients. I prefer to keep it simple. If a recipe looks good but complicated, my first move is to see which ingredients can be spared. If there's a sauce for the meat, but I can make one with jus and a pad of butter in the same pan, I will probably do that instead. If a recipe calls for parsley and cilantro, I may skip the parsley because it is more neutral in flavor and I probably won't miss it. And no way am I making two starches! There's a recipe I love with tofu, broccoli, sweet potatoes, brown rice, and a tahini sauce; I have never once made the rice, as sweet potatoes are quite enough for me. You get the idea. Look for the low-hanging fruit, the thing that won't be missed, and skip it.

5. Buy fresh foods that can be eaten straight from the package.

I dislike and strongly discourage what we call "snack" foods. The vast majority of them are shelf-stable, highly processed foods like breakfast cereal, chips, and "energy bars" made of sugar, flour, and hydrogenated oils that jeopardize your health. I tell clients to avoid them, period.

But in the sense that snacks are simply foods that don't require any work to prepare, well, there are many that I love. Think fresh, whole foods that would spoil if removed from their package or the refrigerator, but, when stored properly, provide convenient nutrition. Olives, apples, cheese, Persian cucumbers, almonds, unsweetened real yogurt, flaxseed crackers, smoked fish...the list goes on. What's great about many of these is they don't spoil quickly, so you can easily keep them on hand for when they're needed.

In the next chapter, you'll learn 50 recipes to make for your eating periods. I know, it seems funny to include recipes in a book on fasting. When I was asked to provide 50 recipes for a book on fasting, I admit I laughed out loud! But with the extra time to focus on making healthy food, you'll enjoy it that much more.

CHAPTER 10

Recipes

MEAT AND FISH

Whole Roast Chicken

When making a roast chicken, always think about prep for other meals. If there's enough meat left on the carcass, pick it over and pull the bits of meat and skin off. Those small pieces and some of the breast meat can be turned into Chicken Salad with Mayo (page 170) or Cobb Salad (page 168). Put the carcass away in a plastic bag in the freezer. When you have enough carcasses, you'll make a Chicken Broth (page 150).

Makes: 4 servings   **Prep time:** 30 minutes to 1 hour
Cook time: 45 minutes to 1 hour

1 whole chicken

sea salt, to taste

1. Take the chicken out of the fridge and remove entirely from its packaging. Rinse the bird only if you notice any off smells or blood on its skin, and pat it dry with paper towels. Sprinkle salt all over the bird, and place it breast side down on a dish. Let come to room temperature on the counter for about 1 hour, depending on the size of the bird. Halfway through, pat the skin dry all around and flip the bird over so that it's breast side up, and preheat the oven to 450°F. Pat it dry again before you put it in the oven.

2. Place the bird on a baking sheet and cook it alone, with nothing else in the oven. The high temperature may produce a lot of smoke, but it'll be worth it for the delicious crispy skin it creates.

3. Check the temperature of the bird at 35 minutes, and remove when it has an internal temperature of about 155°F, after 45 minutes to an hour. Let the bird rest on the counter for at least 20 minutes; it will keep cooking, and the internal temperature will rise to about 165°F. When it's ready, remove the legs, breast, and wings, and reserve any liquid that's collected in the pan. Eat what you want, and put the other pieces, covered with the excess liquid, away in a glass container for a meal another day.

Asian Variation: Before placing the bird in the oven, place once slice of ginger and one garlic clove between each of the leg joints and wing joints. Sprinkle the outside of the bird with 2 tablespoons of soy sauce and the juice of two lemons. Place the lemon rinds inside the cavity, along with another clove of garlic. Cook as directed.

French Dijon Variation: Place two halved lemons and 4 springs of thyme inside the cavity of the bird before cooking. When the chicken is cooked and resting, make the sauce: To a medium skillet over a high flame, add 2 thinly sliced shallots, ¾ cup dry white wine, and ¾ cup of chicken juices from the roasting pan. Reduce the mixture by half, 2 to 3 minutes, add ¼ cup heavy cream, and boil about 1 minute, or until it thickens to the consistency you prefer. Remove the sauce from the heat and whisk in 2 tablespoons of Dijon mustard, 1 tablespoon of minced chives, and salt and pepper to taste. Pour the sauce over the chicken parts assembled on a serving platter or reserve on the side for individual servings.

Chicken Broth

Makes: 2 quarts   **Prep time:** 12 minutes   **Cook time:** 2½ hours

4 roasted chicken carcasses

2 yellow onions,
roughly chopped

2 large carrots,
roughly chopped

2 celery ribs, roughly chopped

1 teaspoon black peppercorn

1 bay leaf

6 sprigs flat-leaf parsley

4 quarts water

1. Combine all of the ingredients in a large stock pot. Bring to a boil, then drop the heat to a medium simmer.

2. Cook for 2½ hours, or until the stock is tasty and well-rounded, and no longer watery. Store in pint or quart containers in the freezer and use it when needed as a base for sauces.

Chicken Livers

Serve these livers with Caramelized Onions (page 176) if you like. Use a fortified wine such as Madeira, port, sherry, or Marsala.

Makes: 2 servings   **Prep time:** 5 minutes   **Cook time:** 5–7 minutes

4 tablespoons butter	¼ cup fortified wine
½ pound chicken livers	½ cup flat-leaf parsley leaves
4 sprigs thyme	sea salt, to taste

1. Heat butter over medium-high in a large frying pan. Once the butter starts foaming, add the salt and chicken livers to the pan and cook for 2 minutes, allowing them to caramelize.

2. Turn the livers over, add the thyme, and cook for an additional minute. Then place the livers on a paper towel–lined plate.

3. Add the fortified wine to the pan, heating just enough to evaporate the alcohol. Stir, removing any caramelized bits on the bottom of the pan, 1 to 2 minutes. When the alcohol is gone, it will no longer burn your nose to smell it. Add salt if needed. Return the livers to the pan to coat with sauce. Garnish with parsley.

Pan-Roasted Rib Eye Steak with Pan Jus

Makes: 2–3 servings   Prep time: 2 minutes active, 45 minutes total   Cook time: 6–20 minutes

1 (1-pound) rib eye steak

4 tablespoons olive oil

½ cup Chicken Broth (page 150)

3 tablespoons room-temperature butter

sea salt, to taste

1. Remove steak from the refrigerator about 45 minutes before cooking, pat it dry, and salt it fully. Flip it over about 20 minutes through, remembering to pat it dry when flipping, and then once more before cooking.

2. Preheat your oven to 200°F, if you wish to cook your steak medium or medium-well. Heat a cast iron skillet or another sturdy pan over a high heat on the stovetop.

3. Add the oil to the pan. Just before it begins to smoke, place the meat in the pan, listening for the searing sound. Leave it there to cook, without moving it, for 3 to 5 minutes. Once the bottom has a nice brown color—you can check by lifting up one edge of the steak to peek at the underside—flip the steak over and do the same on the other side. This will give you a medium-rare steak. If you want to cook it further, place in the oven at 200°F for 5 to 6 minutes for medium, and 7 to 8 minutes for medium-well. When it's done to your liking, remove from the pan and place it on a cutting board to rest for 15 to 20 minutes. Slice and serve.

4. While the steak is resting, make the pan jus. Transfer the pan to the stove top, add the chicken broth, and heat over medium heat, scraping free any pieces stuck to the bottom of the pan. Let liquid reduce by half, 2 to 4 minutes. Then use a whisk or fork to add the butter, 1 tablespoon at a time. Once the butter is incorporated, pour the jus over your meat.

5. If, when you cut into your steak, it's not cooked well enough for you, put it back in the oven for a few more minutes, to your liking.

Pork Belly

Pork belly goes great with Chimichurri sauce (page 196).

Makes: 4 servings   Prep time: 15 minutes active, 12 hours total
Cook time: 1½–2 hours

4–5 pound piece pork belly	4 cups water
2 tablespoons olive oil	sea salt, to taste

1. Place pork on a sheet pan and season generously with salt, then let sit at least 12 hours in the refrigerator after salting, rotating the pork every few hours so the salt is evenly distributed.

2. Preheat oven to 350°F. Set pork belly skin side up on a wire rack set inside a rimmed baking sheet pan. Pour the water into the baking sheet under the pork.

3. Dry the pork skin with a paper towel. Rub the pork skin with oil and season with more salt. Roast for 1½ to 1¾ hours, adding more water to pan as needed, until the skin is golden brown and a thermometer inserted into thickest part reads 195°F to 200°F.

Lamb Meatballs

Makes: 4–5 servings   **Prep time:** 15 minutes
Cook time: 10 minutes

1 pound ground lamb	2 cloves garlic, minced
½ teaspoon ground cumin	1½ teaspoons salt
½ teaspoon ground coriander	1 teaspoon paprika
4 tablespoons fresh cilantro, finely chopped, plus more to serve	½ teaspoon cayenne pepper, or to taste
	4 tablespoons olive oil

1. In a large bowl, combine all ingredients except the oil, and mix until the spices are well incorporated.

2. Shape lamb mixture into medium-sized meatballs, about 1½ inches in diameter. Brush them with oil to grill or broil, or pan fry them in a little oil until well browned all over.

3. Serve with more cilantro, if desired.

Brick Chicken

Makes: 2 servings   **Prep time:** 5 minutes active, 45 minutes total
Cook time: 25–30 minutes

4 chicken thighs, deboned

1 tablespoon olive oil

5–6 sprigs fresh thyme

½ tablespoon unsalted butter

1 clove garlic, crushed, with skin on

sea salt and freshly ground black pepper, to taste

1. Rinse the chicken thighs and pat them dry. Refrigerate uncovered, skin side up, for at least 30 minutes to dry out the skin.

2. Season the chicken with salt and pepper on both sides and place on a paper towel–lined tray for 15 minutes.

3. Heat a large cast iron or nonstick skillet over medium heat and add the oil. Lay all of the chicken thighs in the skillet, skin side down. It's okay if they overlap. Wrap a slightly smaller skillet with foil and place on top of the chicken (this will act as the "brick"), placing 3 to 4 heavy cans in the skillet to weigh it down.

4. Cook the chicken 3 to 5 minutes, then remove the top skillet and check the skin; adjust the heat and rotate the pan as needed so the skin browns evenly. Replace the top skillet and continue to cook until the skin is golden and crisp and the chicken is cooked about three-quarters of the way through, 10 to 12 more minutes.

5. Add the thyme sprigs, butter, and crushed garlic clove. Remove the top skillet and carefully flip the chicken. Cook, uncovered, until the chicken is cooked through, 4 to 6 more minutes. Transfer to a cutting board and let rest 5 minutes. Cut each piece in half to serve.

Pulled Pork

Makes: 6 servings **Prep time:** 20 minutes active, 12–24 hours total **Cook time:** 5-6 hours

1 cup peeled, roughly chopped ginger	¾ cup peeled cloves garlic
1 cup chopped yellow onion	1 (5- to 7-pound) pork roast, preferably shoulder or Boston butt
3 tablespoons paprika	
1 tablespoon Dijon mustard	6 crisp romaine lettuce leaves
½ cup coarse salt	Pickled Red Onions (page 200), to garnish

1. In a blender, blend the ginger, onion, paprika, Dijon mustard, salt, and garlic into a puree. Place the pork into a plastic bag and pour the mixture over the pork; marinate for 12 hours or overnight in the refrigerator. If you can, shift the pork around every few hours to make sure that the marinade is evenly distributed.

2. Preheat the oven to 275°F. Put the pork in a roasting pan and bake for about 5 hours, until it's falling apart and a thermometer inserted into the thickest part reads 170°F.

3. Remove the pork roast from the oven and transfer to a large platter, being careful to save the juices. Allow the meat to rest for about 30 minutes.

4. While still warm, take two forks and shred the meat. Put the shredded pork in a bowl. Pour one quarter of the juice on the shredded pork and mix well to coat. Taste, then add more juice as needed for desired flavor.

5. To serve, spoon the pulled pork mixture onto crisp romaine lettuce leaves. Garnish with pickled onions if you like.

Pan-Seared Salmon Fillet

I don't like to add a sauce to my salmon because I find it's very delicious on its own, but you can add Garlic-Butter-Lemon Sauce (page 192) if you like.

Makes: 3 servings   **Prep time:** 5 minutes active, 35 minutes total   **Cook time:** 12–15 minutes

> 1 large salmon fillet with skin
>
> 3–4 tablespoons olive oil
>
> sea salt, to taste
>
> Dill Cream Sauce, to taste, for serving

1. Season the fish all over with salt and let sit at room temperature, skin side down, for 20 minutes. Pat dry and turn over, letting sit for 10 more minutes.

2. In a large pan over high heat, add the olive oil. Pat the fish very dry with paper towels before cooking. Once ready, place the fillet skin side down and do not move it. Once the skin has browned, 4 to 6 minutes (you can peek at it by lifting up an end while it's cooking), flip the fillet over, and brown the other side. You should have a nice, crispy, almost-sweet crust on the fish. Optionally, served with Dill Cream Sauce.

Dill Cream Sauce: Mix 1 cup mayonnaise, ½ cup crème fraiche, ½ cup sour cream, 2 tablespoons lemon juice, and 3 tablespoons chopped fresh dill in a bowl. Add salt and pepper to taste, and refrigerate until ready to use.

Baked Mackerel

Pair mackerel with Sauce Gribiche (page 193) or Pickled Red Onions (page 200).

Makes: 2 servings   **Prep time:** 10 minutes active, 20 minutes total   **Cook time:** 15 minutes

2 mackerel fillets, bones removed

¼ cup sea salt

1 tablespoon lemon zest

2 tablespoons olive oil

1. Preheat oven to 200°F.

2. Combine the sea salt and lemon in a small bowl. Mix well.

3. Season the mackerel filets using a generous amount of the salt mixture on both sides. Let the seasoned fish sit at room temperature for 10 minutes. Afterward, gently scrape the fish and discard the salt mixture.

4. Lightly brush a sheet pan with olive oil and place the fish, skin side down, on the pan. Roast in oven for 15 minutes or until cooked through; the flesh will no longer be translucent. Fish is delicate, and you're more likely to overcook than undercook it.

Garlic Shrimp

Makes: 2 servings   **Prep time:** 5 minutes active, 20 minutes total   **Cook time:** 2 minutes

8 ounces uncooked large shrimp, peeled, deveined

1 teaspoon coarse salt

¼ cup olive oil

1 tablespoon chopped garlic

1 small bay leaf

1 teaspoon crushed red pepper

1 lemon, zested and cut into wedges

1 tablespoon minced fresh flat-leaf parsley

1. Place shrimp in medium bowl, sprinkle with coarse salt, and toss. Let stand 15 minutes.

2. Heat the oil in a medium skillet over high heat. Add the garlic, bay leaf, and crushed red pepper, and stir for 1 minute.

3. Add shrimp to the skillet, laying them flat on one side to cook for 30 seconds to 1 minute, then flip the shrimp and cook for an additional 30 seconds. Remove from heat and add 1 teaspoon of lemon zest.

4. Transfer the shrimp to a serving dish. Garnish with parsley and lemon wedges.

HEARTY DISHES

Bacon and Kale

This is my favorite breakfast on days when I eat it, which is rare! I love this dish on its own and have never felt the need for bread or potatoes. If I'm in the mood I'll add a fried egg, and sometimes I add pickled vegetables or squeeze lemon on the kale if I want a bright or acidic element.

Makes: 1 serving   **Prep time:** 3 minutes   **Cook time:** 10 minutes

4 slices bacon

half bunch of kale, de-stemmed

sea salt, to taste

1. Put a cast iron skillet or another sturdy pan over a high heat, and get it very hot. Wet your hand and flick water onto the pan to make sure it sizzles; if not, wait until it's hotter.

2. When ready, evenly place the bacon slices in the pan. While you're waiting for them to cook you can cut the leaves of kale into smaller pieces, or just rip them in half, or skip this step altogether (I do).

3. When the bacon starts to curl at the edges, turn it over and cook until it's as crispy as you like it, 3 to 5 minutes. Place on a paper towel or cooling rack to cool.

4. As soon as the bacon is removed, add the kale to the pan with the bacon fat while it's still hot. Add salt and sauté until soft, about 3 minutes. Season with salt.

5. Pile the kale on a plate and add the bacon strips on top.

Slow Baked Beans with Mustard Greens

I made this dish one year for Thanksgiving and it was a hit. It cooked all day, and got better as the hours passed. Save it for a cold day when you'll be home for a long while and won't mind having the oven on. It's adapted from the *New York Times* Cooking section, and it has my "simplify and skip hard steps" approach all over it. You can use any hearty greens in this recipe, but I like to use mustard greens.

Makes: 10 servings   **Prep time:** 30 minutes   **Cook time:** 4–6 hours

4 sprigs fresh flat-leaf parsley

2 sprigs fresh thyme

1 bay leaf

½ cup olive oil, pork fat, or other fat for sautéing the vegetables

2 onions, roughly chopped

3 carrots, roughly chopped

4 cloves garlic, roughly chopped

1 (6-ounce) can tomato paste, dissolved in 1 cup water

1½ cups white beans, soaked overnight, drained and rinsed

5 cups water, plus more as needed

3 bunches mustard greens, de-stemmed, leaves halved

1 ham hock or 1–2 large chunks slab bacon

sea salt, to taste

freshly ground black pepper, to taste

1. Preheat the oven to 225°F.

2. Make a bouquet garni by wrapping the parsley, thyme, and bay leaf together with a string. This will be removed at the end of cooking.

3. In a 3 to 4-quart pot over medium heat, sauté the onions and carrots in the oil or fat. When the onion is soft, about 5 minutes, add the garlic and sauté another 30 seconds. Then stir in the dissolved tomato paste and bring to a simmer. Add the drained beans and the 5 cups of water, the bouquet garni, and salt and pepper. Bring to a simmer.

4. Transfer to a large baking dish, and add the mustard greens and ham hocks or bacon slabs. Bake for 3 to 4 hours, folding the beans every hour to bring those on the bottom up to the top. If the beans on the bottom are dry and not yet fully cooked, then add more water ½ cup at a time. Taste each time and add salt if needed.

5. Remove from the oven when the beans are creamy and the dish has a sweetness to it. If the beans don't soften after 2 hours of cooking, raise the temperature of the oven to 300°F and continue cooking. Once done, let cool somewhat and remove the bouquet garni before serving.

Chicken Curry

2 pounds boneless, skinless chicken breasts or thighs, cut into 1-inch cubes

1½ tablespoons sea salt

2½ teaspoons mild curry powder

2 tablespoons coconut or olive oil

1 (14-ounce) can full-fat coconut milk

1 (2½-inch) piece ginger, peeled and sliced

4 cloves garlic

½ medium onion, chopped

2 cups broccoli florets

4 cups baby spinach leaves

zest of 1 lime

cilantro leaves with tender stems, to garnish

1. Toss the chicken with salt in a medium bowl and let sit for 10 minutes, then add curry powder. Meanwhile, purée the coconut milk, ginger, and garlic in a blender until very smooth.

2. Heat the oil in a large skillet over medium-high heat. Add the onion and stir until softened, about 4 minutes.

3. Add the chicken and the coconut milk mixture to skillet and cook, tossing occasionally, until chicken is cooked through and sauce has thickened, 7 to 10 minutes.

4. Add broccoli florets to the skillet and cook until bright green in color, about 1 minute, then add the spinach and the lime zest. Top with cilantro.

Parmesan and Herb Frittata

Makes: 6 servings   **Prep time:** 12 minutes   **Cook time:** 10–15 minutes

2 teaspoons extra-virgin olive oil

1 teaspoon minced garlic

1 large sweet onion, chopped

12 large eggs

1 tablespoon salt, divided, plus more to taste

1 cup grated Parmesan cheese

½ cup chopped fresh flat-leaf parsley

½ cup sliced fresh basil

¼ teaspoon freshly ground black pepper

3 tablespoons heavy cream

1. Preheat oven to 350°F.

2. Add oil to a skillet on medium heat and cook the garlic and onion together, along with ½ tablespoon of the salt.

2. In a bowl, whisk together the eggs, cheese, parsley, basil, the remaining ½ tablespoon salt, pepper, and heavy cream.

3. When the onion and garlic are cooked through, about 2 minutes, add the egg mixture to the skillet, stirring occasionally, as you want your eggs to cook evenly. Once the egg mixture starts become thicker and some of the eggs are cooked, 2 to 3 minutes, place the skillet of eggs into the oven, and cook for 5 to 7 minutes or until the center of the frittata is firm.

SALADS

Cobb Salad

This is a go-to at many restaurants when I'm looking for something fat- and vegetable-rich. It's equally delicious with either Bibb or romaine lettuce.

Makes: 2 servings **Prep time:** 12 minutes **Cook time:** 8 minutes

1 hard-boiled egg, sliced

1 avocado, halved and sliced

½ cup sliced cherry tomatoes (optional)

1 cup cubed or shredded chicken breast

3 to 4 slices of cooked, chopped bacon

¼ cup crumbled blue cheese

2 tablespoons sliced green onions (optional)

1 head of lettuce, leaves separated

olive oil, to taste

lemon juice, to taste

1. In a large bowl, toss together the egg, avocado, tomatoes, if using, chicken, bacon, blue cheese, and green onions, if using. Place on top of the lettuce.

2. Drizzle with olive oil and lemon juice to taste, or use any salad dressing you like.

Zesty Coleslaw

Makes: 6 servings   **Prep time:** 10 minutes active, 25 minutes total

1 head green cabbage, thinly sliced

zest of 3 limes

juice of 6 limes

1 bunch cilantro, chopped

1 tablespoon sea salt, plus more as needed

2 tablespoons olive oil

1. Place the cabbage in a large bowl. Add the sea salt and squeeze the cabbage pieces well, until they are no longer stiff, and set aside for 15 minutes. Then, drain the juice from the cut cabbage and discard.

2. Add the lime zest, juice, and cilantro to the cabbage. Taste, add salt as needed, and place in the fridge. When ready to serve, add the olive oil and toss lightly.

Chicken Salad with Mayo

I like to use the leftover chicken breast from a roast chicken in this salad. If you prefer not to use buttermilk in this recipe, use ½ cup mayonnaise. This recipe has a strong mustard flavor, so you can use less if you're not a big fan of mustard.

Makes: 8 servings   **Prep time:** 10 minutes

¼ cup buttermilk (optional)

½ clove minced garlic

¼ cup Mayonnaise (page 187)

2 tablespoons Dijon mustard

1 tablespoon lemon juice

1 teaspoon lemon zest

½ teaspoon Tabasco sauce

4 cups shredded roasted chicken

1 celery rib, diced

¼ cup diced red onion

¼ cup roughly chopped flat-leaf parsley

sea salt, to taste

freshly ground black pepper, to taste

Mix the buttermilk, if using, garlic, mayonnaise, mustard, lemon zest, lemon juice, and Tabasco in a large bowl until well combined. Add the chicken and remaining ingredients to the mixture, mix again, and taste to adjust the seasoning.

Kale Salad with Roasted Pumpkin Seeds

Makes: 4 servings   **Prep time:** 30 minutes   **Cook time:** 10 minutes

½ cup pumpkin seeds

¼ to ⅓ cup extra-virgin olive oil, divided

¼ teaspoon ground cumin

¼ teaspoon cayenne pepper

1 bunch lacinato or curly kale, de-stemmed, sliced into ribbons

zest of 1 lemon

juice of 2 lemons

½ cup grated Parmesan cheese

sea salt, to taste

1. Preheat the oven to 200°F.

2. Mix pumpkin seeds in a bowl with 1 tablespoon of olive oil and the cumin and cayenne. Roast the seeds on baking sheet for about 10 minutes, or until they are toasted, being careful not to let them burn. Alternatively, roast them in a pan on the stove over low to medium heat if you feel you have more control that way.

3. In a large bowl, mix the kale with the lemon zest. Add the lemon juice, massaging the kale leaves to soften them. Mix in the remaining olive oil, and then the cheese. Finish with salt to taste, and top with toasted pumpkin seeds.

Tomato and Sardine Lettuce Wrap

Makes: 4 servings   **Prep time:** 10 minutes active, 30 minutes total   **Cook time:** 12-15 minutes

4 tablespoons olive oil, plus more to taste

4 cloves garlic, sliced

2 cups halved cherry tomatoes

1 teaspoon lemon zest

2 (4-ounce) cans sardines, packed in oil, drained

flat-leaf parsley, chopped, to taste

fresh sweet basil, chopped, to taste

lemon juice, to taste

4 small romaine leaves, from near the heart

sea salt, to taste

freshly ground black pepper, to taste

1. In a large skillet over medium heat, add olive oil and cook garlic, stirring often until garlic is soft, about 2 minutes. Add the tomatoes; season with salt and pepper and cook, stirring occasionally, until falling apart, 8 to 10 minutes.

2. Once the tomatoes are cooked, add lemon zest and chill in the fridge until cold, about 20 minutes.

3. When the tomatoes are cold, mix them with the drained sardines, breaking up the fillets. Add chopped herbs, olive oil, and lemon juice to your preference.

4. Separate the leaves from the romaine hearts and add the sardine and tomato mixture to each leaf. Serve like a taco.

Seaweed Salad

Eat this as a starter to any meal, or an accompaniment to an Asian dish.

Makes: 2 servings   **Prep time:** 10 minutes

3 tablespoons rice vinegar

3 tablespoons soy sauce

2 tablespoons sesame oil

1 teaspoon finely grated peeled fresh ginger

½ teaspoon minced garlic

½ cup wakame seaweed, soaked, drained, and cut into ½-inch-wide strips

2 scallions, thinly sliced

1 tablespoon toasted sesame seeds (optional)

Stir together the vinegar, soy sauce, sesame oil, ginger, and garlic in a medium bowl and let sit for 1 to 2 minutes. Combine the liquid with the seaweed and scallions. Sprinkle salad with sesame seeds.

VEGETABLES

Roasted Sunchokes

Makes: 3 servings   Prep time: 5 minutes   Cook time: 30 minutes

10-12 sunchokes, halved, scrubbed very well to remove all debris

½ cup olive oil

¼ cup butter

4 sprigs fresh thyme

sea salt, to taste

1. Place the sunchokes in a medium pot with cold water at high heat. Once the water comes to a boil, add salt and turn down to a low simmer. Cook the sunchokes until they are soft, about 15 minutes, then dry them on a towel and place in the fridge.

2. When the sunchokes are cool, heat the oil in a pan over medium-high heat. When the oil is hot, place the sunchokes flesh side down, turn the heat to medium, and allow them to caramelize. Cook them slowly, making sure to not move them around, but it is OK to check them, gently lifting them to see the color underneath. Cook until the flesh is golden brown, about 10 minutes.

3. When they have good color, add the butter and thyme, and cook until the butter stops foaming, about 2 minutes. Then add salt to taste.

Caramelized Onions

Caramelized onions are a great topping to many foods—I find them especially good on chicken, steak, or hummus.

Makes: 6 servings   **Prep time:** 5 minutes   **Cook time:** 45 minutes

4 tablespoons olive oil

2 large sweet yellow onions, cut into ¼-inch strips

1 cup water, divided

sea salt, to taste

1. Heat the oil in pan over medium heat and add the cut onions, mixing well to coat them with the oil. Cover the pan with a lid.

2. Once the onions begin to soften, about 2 minutes, add ½ cup of the water and continue cooking on high heat with the lid on. Stir every 3 minutes. When the onions are cooked through, turn the heat down to medium and remove the lid.

3. Allow the onions to caramelize while constantly stirring them; if they get too dark or begin to burn, add a little more water and stir again. The process should take 30 to 40 minutes. Once the onions are brown deep in color, add salt to taste.

Sautéed Broccoli Rabe or Broccolini

Makes: 2 servings   **Prep time:** 5 minutes   **Cook time:** 10 minutes

1 bunch broccoli rabe or 2 bunches broccolini, stems trimmed, roughly chopped

6 tablespoons olive oil

1 teaspoon crushed red pepper

4 tablespoons grated Parmesan cheese (optional)

sea salt, to taste

Heat olive oil in a large skillet over high heat, add the broccoli rabe or broccolini, and turn heat down to medium. Sauté for 4 to 5 minutes or until the greens have softened and the leafy parts are wilted, adding salt, crushed red pepper, and Parmesan, if using, toward the end.

Cauliflower Soup

Makes: 3 servings   **Prep time:** 15 minutes   **Cook time:** 20 minutes

1½ cups olive oil, divided

½ head of cauliflower, cut into ½-inch pieces

1 clove garlic, minced

1 small shallot, minced

1-3 cups water, divided

sherry vinegar, to taste (optional)

sea salt, to taste

1. Heat ½ cup of the oil in a frying pan over medium heat. Once the oil is hot, add the cauliflower and season with salt, cooking until it is light brown, about 5 minutes.

2. Remove the cauliflower and set aside, leaving the oil in the pan. Add garlic to the warm oil and cook until it is golden brown, less than 1 minute, then add the shallots and a little salt, stirring frequently until the shallots are soft, 1 to 2 minutes.

3. Add the cauliflower back to the pan along with 1 cup of the water and cover with a lid. Cook the mixture until the cauliflower is soft, 7 to 8 minutes. If the liquid evaporates before the cauliflower is soft, add more water, ½ cup at a time, to finish cooking.

4. Transfer cauliflower to a blender. Blend at a slow speed, adding the remaining olive oil at a slow drizzle while the blender is on. Once all the oil has been mixed into the soup, blend on high until smooth. Turn blender off, taste, and add salt if needed. Just before serving, add a dash of sherry vinegar to finish off the soup, if desired.

Mushroom Cream Soup

Makes: 4 servings   **Prep time:** 15 minutes   **Cook time:** 30 minutes

4 cloves garlic, minced

1 cup minced yellow onion

¼ cup butter

2 pounds cremini and shiitake mushrooms, cut into strips

½ cup dry white wine

1 cup chicken stock

2½ cups whole milk

2½ cups heavy cream

5 sprigs fresh thyme

1 bay leaf

sea salt, to taste

1. In a medium, heavy-bottomed pot, cook the garlic and onions in the butter over medium-low heat until the onions are translucent, then add mushrooms and salt, and cook for 5 minutes.

2. Continue cooking until all of the juices have been cooked out, then add the wine and cook until the alcohol has boiled off (approximately 2 minutes; the liquid should smell good and should not burn your nose).

3. Add the chicken stock, cooking it down by half, 10 to 12 minutes. Then, add the milk and cream, along with the thyme and bay leaf, and lower the heat to medium-low heat. Simmer the soup for 10 minutes while stirring, until all the flavors come together.

4. Strain the soup to separate the onion, garlic, mushrooms, and herbs from the liquid, reserving the liquid. Add the vegetables to a blender with a small amount of the liquid. Blend until smooth, adding the liquid a little at a time until all the liquid is incorporated, and serve.

Roasted Kabocha Squash

Makes: 6 servings   **Prep time:** 10 minutes   **Cook time:** 45 minutes

  1 kabocha squash, cut into 1-inch strips

  3–4 tablespoons coconut oil

  sea salt, to taste

1. Preheat oven to 375°F.

2. Toss the squash pieces in the coconut oil and season with salt.

3. Place pieces neatly in a glass baking dish, making sure that the flesh touches the bottom of the dish. If it's too crowded, use a second dish. Bake for about 45 minutes or until soft.

Smoky-Spicy Variation: Make a chipotle butter by blending 1 stick of room-temperature butter with 1 teaspoon of chipotle powder and a pinch of salt. Place a dollop of butter onto each slice of squash while still warm.

Fresh Variation: Mix 2 tablespoons tahini with ½ cup whole-milk strained yogurt, and spread the mixture on a serving platter. In a medium bowl, make a dressing by whisking together 2 tablespoons lemon or lime juice, 1 teaspoon honey, ¼ teaspoon cayenne pepper, ½ teaspoon salt, and 3 tablespoons olive oil. Place the squash slices, once cooled, on the yogurt spread and top with the dressing. Top with 1 cup of chopped mint.

Buttered Leeks

Makes: 6 servings   Prep time: 15 minutes   Cook time: 25 minutes

¼ cup dry white wine

½ cup chicken stock, plus more as needed

6 leeks, white part only, cleaned thoroughly to remove any dirt or grit

½ pound butter

½ teaspoon lemon or orange zest

sea salt, to taste

1. To a medium sauce pan over medium-high heat, add the wine, cooking off the alcohol. Then add the chicken stock, leeks, salt, and butter. Make sure that the leeks are under the liquid level, and add more chicken stock if needed.

2. Bring ingredients to a low simmer and cover with a lid. Cook the leeks until they are medium soft, 12 to 15 minutes, then remove and place them on a serving dish. Reduce the liquid by half, about 5 minutes.

3. Turn off the heat and add the lemon or orange zest. Once leeks have cooled to room temperature, about 5 minutes, cut them in half lengthwise. Place cut side down on a plate and cover with the sauce from the pot.

Creamed Spinach

Makes: 2 servings   **Prep time:** 10 minutes   **Cook time:** 20–25 minutes

6 cups fresh, cleaned, and dried spinach leaves

3 tablespoons unsalted butter

2 tablespoons olive oil

1 small sweet onion, minced

3 cloves garlic, minced

¾ cup heavy cream

¼ cup grated Parmesan cheese

sea salt, to taste

freshly ground black pepper, to taste

1. Bring a medium pot of water to a boil over high heat. Blanch the spinach for 10 to 15 seconds in salted water and then place in an ice water bath for 30 seconds. Drain, and squeeze out the excess water. Chop the cooked spinach into small pieces.

2. Heat the butter and oil in a large skillet over medium-high heat and add the minced onion and garlic. Cook, stirring frequently, until soft, 3 to 4 minutes.

3. Add the cream and cook until it reduces by half, about 10 minutes. Then add the Parmesan and season with salt and pepper to taste, stirring frequently until the cheese has melted. Add spinach and cook until it's hot, about 5 more minutes. Serve immediately.

Cauliflower Mash

Makes: 4 servings   **Prep time:** 12 minutes   **Cook time:** 6 minutes

1 head cauliflower

2 tablespoons olive oil

1 clove garlic, minced

2 tablespoons chopped
fresh rosemary

2 tablespoons butter

2 tablespoons heavy cream

sea salt, to taste

1. Prepare a steamer basket over 4 inches of water in a pot, and bring to a boil. Break the cauliflower into florets and add them to the steamer basket over the boiling water. Allow to steam for 1 minute uncovered, then cover the pot and steam until soft, about 3 minutes more.

2. Heat olive oil in a skillet over medium-low heat and add chopped rosemary and garlic, cooking 1 to 2 minutes. Add butter and melt, and add cauliflower to coat with seasoning. Cook 1 more minute.

3. Mash cauliflower with a potato masher in the skillet. Pour contents of skillet into blender, and add heavy cream while blending. Add salt while blending. Serve like mashed potatoes.

Roasted Cauliflower

A common mistake when roasting cauliflower is to not roast it long enough; a longer roast will produce more caramelization and a tastier end product. For the same reason, do not move the florets during the cooking process. Serve with Tahini Dressing (page 190), if you'd like.

Makes: 2 servings   **Prep time:** 8 minutes   **Cook time:** 45 minutes

  1 head cauliflower

  4 tablespoons olive oil

  sea salt, to taste

1. Preheat oven to 375°F.

2. Break the cauliflower into florets and toss in a large mixing bowl with olive oil and salt.

3. Spread on a baking sheet and bake in the oven for 30 to 45 minutes, or until well caramelized.

Spicy Variation: Add the following into the mixing bowl when coating the cauliflower with oil: 2 tablespoons minced garlic, 1 teaspoon cumin, 1 teaspoon paprika, ½ teaspoon turmeric, and ¼ teaspoon cayenne pepper.

Mushrooms Sautéed in Butter and Thyme

Makes: 4 servings   **Prep time:** 10 minutes   **Cook time:** 15 minutes

3 cloves garlic, minced, divided

½ cup chopped fresh flat-leaf parsley leaves, plus more for garnish

4–5 cups fresh wild mushrooms, roughly chopped

5–6 tablespoons olive oil, divided

½ teaspoon coarse sea salt

3 tablespoon butter

3 sprigs fresh thyme

1 tablespoon lemon juice

freshly ground black pepper, to taste

1. Mix one-third of the minced garlic with the chopped parsley, and set aside.

2. Place mushrooms in a large bowl and coat with 2 tablespoons of the olive oil. Add in the remaining garlic and salt, and mix well.

3. Heat 2 to 3 tablespoons of the olive oil in large heavy skillet over medium-high heat. Add mushroom mixture and sauté. If the mushrooms appear dry and start sticking to the pan, add 1 or 2 more tablespoons of olive oil. Cook until mushrooms are brown and just tender, about 6 minutes. Add butter and thyme and allow the mushrooms to cook for 5 minutes.

4. Remove skillet from heat. Mix in parsley mixture and lemon juice. Season to taste with salt and pepper and garnish with additional fresh parsley if you like.

SAUCES, DRESSINGS, AND CONDIMENTS

Mayonnaise

Makes: ½ cup   **Prep time:** 12 minutes

1 egg yolk

¾ cup olive oil, divided

1 teaspoon apple
cider vinegar

½ teaspoon lemon juice

sea salt, to taste

1. Place egg yolk in small bowl with a pinch of salt, and whisk while adding the olive oil in a slow drizzle.

2. Once half of the olive oil has combined with the egg yolk, add the vinegar and the lemon juice and mix well.

3. Drizzle in the other half of the olive oil, mixing well until all of the ingredients are emulsified. Add salt to taste, mix briefly again, and refrigerate for up to 2 weeks.

Garlic Aioli Variation: Mash two cloves of garlic into a smooth paste with a mortar and pestle; if you don't have one, you can mince the garlic very finely. Place half the garlic paste in a small bowl with the egg yolk, and whisk together with a pinch of salt before beginning to incorporate the oil as described in step 1. Follow the recipe and taste at the end, adding more of the garlic paste to your preference.

Smoked Paprika Variation: Add ¼ teaspoon of smoked paprika to the finished mayonnaise, adding more, ¼ teaspoon at a time, to taste.

Guacamole

juice of 2 limes, divided

2 ripe avocados, mashed

2 tablespoons chopped onion

1 jalapeno, minced

4 tablespoons chopped fresh cilantro

sea salt, to taste

Squeeze half of the lime juice over the avocados and sprinkle with a dash of salt, then mash thoroughly. Fold in the chopped onion, jalapeno, and cilantro. Mix and salt to taste. Squeeze a bit more lime on top to help the guacamole hold its color.

Olive Tapenade

Tapenade can be used as a sauce or condiment for any protein dish, or as a dip for vegetables.

Makes: 12 servings   **Prep time:** 8 minutes

2 cups pitted olives

1 teaspoon lemon zest

1 tablespoon lemon juice

2 tablespoons flat-leaf parsley, chopped

1 clove garlic, chopped

½ anchovy fillet, chopped

Place the olives in a food processor and pulse until they are chopped very small, but before they become pureed, then add them to a bowl. Add the lemon zest, lemon juice, parsley, garlic, and anchovy to the olive mixture. Mix well and store in refrigerator.

Tahini Dressing

This recipe is about as simple as it gets! Tahini is a great sauce for roasted vegetables as it gives a nutty, earthy flavor.

Makes: 6 servings   **Prep time:** 5 minutes

⅓ cup tahini

⅓ cup water

¼ cup lemon juice

2 cloves garlic, chopped

½ teaspoon honey

sea salt, to taste

Blend all ingredients in a blender until smooth.

Avocado Dressing

Makes: 4 servings   **Prep time:** 5 minutes

1 ripe avocado

2 tablespoons apple cider vinegar

1 tablespoon lime juice

1 cup olive oil

sea salt, to taste

freshly ground black pepper, to taste

Blend avocado, vinegar, lime juice, salt, and pepper in a food processor until the ingredients are creamy, then turn the food processor to low (if your machine has multiple speeds), or pulse, while slowly adding the olive oil until all is blended. Chill in the fridge and store for up to 1 week.

Easy Balsamic Dressing

I make this dressing in batches and use it for just about every salad I make simply because it's easy and available. Choose whichever herbs you like best for this recipe; I like to use dried oregano or thyme.

Makes: 8 servings   **Prep time:** 5 minutes

1 tablespoon Dijon mustard

⅓ cup balsamic vinegar

1 teaspoon dried herbs

⅔ cup olive oil

½ teaspoon salt

Whisk together the mustard, vinegar, salt, and herbs. Add the oil a little at a time, whisking to emulsify. If you like a thick dressing that will not separate while storing, then use a blender. For a lighter texture, hand whisk.

Garlic-Butter-Lemon Sauce

This sauce pairs extremely well with salmon.

Makes: 4 servings   **Prep time:** 2 minutes   **Cook time:** 5–6 minutes

4 tablespoons unsalted
butter, divided

2 cloves garlic, minced

¼ cup chicken broth

2 tablespoons lemon juice

1. In a small saucepan, melt 1 tablespoon butter over medium heat. Add garlic and sauté until lightly golden brown, about 1 to 2 minutes.

2. Pour in chicken broth and lemon juice. Let sauce simmer until it has reduced by half, about 3 minutes. Stir in remaining butter and whisk until combined. Serve immediately.

Sauce Gribiche

Sauce gribiche goes well on top of fish, meat, or vegetables.

Makes: 4 servings   **Prep time:** 5 minutes   **Cook time:** 12 minutes

- 1 tablespoon Dijon mustard
- 1 tablespoon white wine vinegar
- 3 tablespoons olive oil
- 1 tablespoon capers
- 2 cornichons, finely chopped
- 1 hard-boiled egg, finely chopped
- sea salt, to taste
- 1 tablespoon chopped parsley
- freshly ground black pepper, to taste

Mix everything except the parsley in a bowl and adjust seasoning to taste. Stir in parsley just before serving.

Tomatillo Salsa

Tomatillo salsa goes great on eggs, fish, and pork.

Makes: 8 servings   **Prep time:** 8 minutes   **Cook time:** 10 minutes

5–6 medium tomatillos, husked and rinsed

¼ cup chopped white or yellow onion

2 serrano peppers or 1 jalapeno, stemmed

1 bunch fresh cilantro, roughly chopped, thick stems removed

¼ cup water

sea salt, to taste

1. Preheat a broiler.

2. Roast the tomatillos, onion, and peppers on a baking sheet 4 inches below a very hot broiler until well roasted, about 8 minutes.

3. In a blender or food processor, combine the tomatillos, onion, and peppers, including all the juice that has run onto the baking sheet. Add the cilantro and water, blend to a coarse puree, and transfer to a serving dish. Season with a generous amount of salt.

Asian Dipping Sauce

Serve as a dipping sauce for meat or a glaze for vegetables. Use mild versions of soy sauce and olive oil to allow the other flavors to stand out.

Makes: 8–10 servings   **Prep time:** 5 minutes   **Cook time:** 3 minutes

2 medium cloves garlic, minced

½ cup light or low-sodium soy sauce

¼ cup rice wine vinegar

2 tablespoons finely grated fresh ginger

2 tablespoons chopped green onion

1 teaspoon sugar

1 teaspoon sesame oil

½ tablespoon light olive oil

Roast garlic in a pan with olive oil over medium heat until golden brown, just about 1 minute. Then add all of the ingredients to the pan, remove from the heat, and stir well. Combine everything in a lidded jar, and shake well.

Chimichurri

Chimichurri is a great accompaniment to steak.

Makes: 8–10 servings   **Prep time:** 10 minutes

½ cup red wine vinegar

1 teaspoon sea salt, plus more to taste

3–4 cloves garlic, thinly sliced or minced

1 Fresno chile or red jalapeno, finely chopped

½ cup minced fresh cilantro

¼ cup minced fresh flat-leaf parsley

¾ cup extra-virgin olive oil

1. Combine vinegar, salt, garlic, and chile in a medium bowl and let stand for 10 minutes.

2. Stir in cilantro and parsley. Using a fork, whisk in the oil. Adjust salt to taste.

Pesto

In my opinion, pesto goes well on just about anything, especially noodles (including no-carb shirataki noodles), fish, and chicken. It brings a bright, fresh, basil flavor to your dish. You can store pesto in a clean ice cube tray and defrost individual cubes when you want to use them.

Makes: 4–6 servings   **Prep time:** 15 minutes

4 loosely packed cups fresh basil leaves

½ cup grated Parmesan cheese

⅓ cup pine nuts or walnuts

3 cloves garlic, minced

¾ cup olive oil, plus more as needed

sea salt, to taste

freshly ground black pepper, to taste

1. Pulse basil and nuts in a food processor until homogeneous. Add the cheese and garlic, and pulse until combined.

2. Slowly drizzle in the olive oil while the processor is running on low speed if your machine has multiple speeds, otherwise, add 1 to 2 tablespoons of oil at a time and check consistency before adding more. Once the oil is completely combined and the pesto is the consistency you want, mix in the salt and pepper.

Tomato Sauce

Makes: 8 servings   **Prep time:** 5 minutes   **Cook time:** 30–35 minutes

4 cloves garlic, sliced

¼ cup olive oil

2 (16-ounce) cans whole or diced tomatoes

½ teaspoon sugar (optional)

½ cup fresh chopped basil

sea salt, to taste

freshly ground black pepper, to taste

1. In a large skillet over medium-high heat, brown the garlic in the oil, just under 1 minute.

2. Add the tomatoes and season with salt and pepper. Simmer, cooking until the sauce has thickened to desired consistency, 20 to 30 minutes.

3. Taste, and adjust seasoning. If it's too acidic, add the sugar and mix well, then taste again. Stir in chopped basil and serve with vegetable of your choice.

Pickling Liquid Base

You can pickle any vegetable you want in this liquid—cauliflower, string beans, carrots, turnips, or whatever is lying around. Just place the vegetable in a jar, pour in enough pickling liquid to cover them completely, and store in the refrigerator until they are ready. They'll turn more vinegary over time.

Makes: about 2 portions, but you can reuse the liquid once the pickles are gone   **Prep time:** 3 minutes active, 24 hours total
Cook time: 10 minutes

1 cup water

½ cup rice wine vinegar

4 tablespoons sugar

1 teaspoon sea salt

Combine the water, rice wine vinegar, sugar, and salt in a medium pot, and bring to a boil. Let cool and wait 24 hours before using.

Pickled Red Onions

Pickled onions go great with pork dishes and hamburgers.

Makes: 20 servings **Prep time:** 10 minutes active, 48 hours total **Cook time:** 10 minutes

2 cups water	2 teaspoons sea salt
1¼ cup red wine or apple cider vinegar	3 red onions, sliced into thin rings
½ cup sugar	1 teaspoon freshly ground black pepper

1. Place the water, vinegar, sugar, and salt in a pot and bring to a boil.

2. Place the onions in a large glass pickling jar set in the sink, in case of spills. Season the onions with black pepper, pour in the pickling liquid, and let them cool at room temperature. Then cover and place in the refrigerator for at least 48 hours before using.

Acknowledgments

To Tim: You have Michelin-star taste buds and a love for my Sephardic home cooking. What more could I want? We all know the recipes in this book really belong to you. Someday, I'll help you write your own.

To the readers of my first book who wrote to me with stories of your success: Thank you. It's because of you that I found the motivation to write another one.

To MB: How many diet books have you helped usher into the world now? Count me among the grateful authors.

And to Hadim, who coached me through those long hot summer days in NYC during my first intermittent fast, and opened my eyes to the possibility of a lifetime practice.

About the Author

Kristen Mancinelli, MS, RDN, is a registered dietitian nutritionist specializing in high-fat/low-carb and ketogenic diets and intermittent fasting. She guides clients to success using practical strategies that make sense for their busy lives. Kristen has over 12 years of experience in nutrition counseling, helping adults of all ages lose weight and prevent or manage insulin resistance and related conditions. In addition, she has experience in digital health technology, healthcare and social marketing, and public health communications and advocacy. She holds a bachelor's degree in chemistry from NYU and a master's in nutrition and public health from Columbia University. Reach her with questions and for support at www .kristenmancinelli.com.